CONCEPTUAL
MODELS
OF NURSING

Global Perspectives

CONCEPTUAL MODELS OF NURSING

Global Perspectives

FIFTH EDITION

Joyce J. Fitzpatrick
Elizabeth Brooks Ford Professor and Dean
Frances Payne Bolton School of Nursing
Case Western Reserve University
Cleveland, Ohio

Ann L. Whall
Professor, School of Nursing
Associate Director, The Geriatrics Center
The University of Michigan
Ann Arbor, Michigan

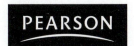

Boston   Columbus   Indianapolis   New York   San Francisco
Amsterdam   Cape Town   Dubai   London   Madrid   Milan   Munich   Paris   Montreal   Toronto
Delhi   Mexico City   São Paulo   Sydney   Hong Kong   Seoul   Singapore   Taipei Tokyo

Publisher: Julie Levin Alexander
Publisher's Assistant: Sarah Henrich
Executive Editor: Pamela Fuller
Development Editor: Nicole Coady
Editorial Assistant: Erin Sullivan
Project Manager: Cathy O'Connell
Program Manager: Erin Rafferty
Director, Product Management Services: Etain O'Dea
Team Lead, Program Management: Melissa Bashe
Team Lead, Project Management: Cynthia Zonneveld
Full-Service Project Manager: Patty Donovan, SPi Global
Manufacturing Buyer: Maura Zaldivar-Garcia

Art Director: Diane Ernsberger
Cover Design: Cenveo/Nesbitt
Vice President of Sales & Marketing: David Gesell
Vice President, Director of Marketing: Margaret Waples
Senior Product Marketing Manager: Phoenix Harvey
Field Marketing Manager: Debi Doyle
Marketing Specialist: Michael Sirinides
Marketing Assistant: Amy Pfund
Media Project Manager: Lisa Rinaldi
Composition: SPi Global
Printer/Binder: RR Donnelley/STP Harrisonburg
Cover Printer: RR Donnelley/STP Harrisonburg
Cover Image: Maxx-Studio/Shutterstock

Credits and acknowledgments borrowed from other sources and reproduced, with permission, in this textbook appear on the appropriate page within text.

Notice: Care has been taken to confirm the accuracy of information presented in this book. The authors, editors, and the publisher, however, cannot accept any responsibility for errors or omissions or for consequences from application of the information in this book and make no warranty, express or implied, with respect to its contents.

The authors and publisher have exerted every effort to ensure that drug selections and dosages set forth in this text are in accord with current recommendations and practice at time of publication. However, in view of ongoing research, changes in government regulations, and the constant flow of information relating to drug therapy and drug reactions, the reader is urged to check the package inserts of all drugs for any change in indications of dosage and for added warnings and precautions. This is particularly important when the recommended agent is a new and/or infrequently employed drug.

Library of Congress Cataloging-in-Publication Data

Conceptual models of nursing. Global perspectives / [edited by] Joyce J. Fitzpatrick, Ann L. Whall. — Fifth edition.
    p. ; cm.
    Global perspectives
    Preceded by Conceptual models of nursing : analysis and application / [edited by] Joyce J. Fitzpatrick, Ann L. Whall. 4th ed. c2005.
    ISBN 978-0-13-380575-8 — ISBN 0-13-380575-1
    I. Fitzpatrick, Joyce J., editor. II. Whall, Ann L., editor. III. Title: International imperatives.
    [DNLM: 1. Models, Nursing. 2. Philosophy, Nursing. WY 20.5]
    RT84.5
    610.7301—dc23   2015017035

10 9 8 7 6 5 4 3 2 1

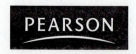

ISBN-13: 978-0-13-380575-8
ISBN-10: 0-13-380575-1

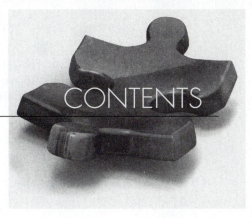

CONTENTS

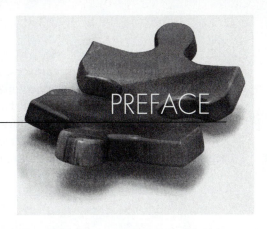

PREFACE

This fifth edition of *Conceptual Models of Nursing* is a testament to the power of nursing knowledge development globally, and the concomitant care being provided in many settings throughout the world. Nurse scholars from several countries share their intellectual pursuits and describe their efforts to delineate the theoretical rationale behind the exemplary care that is provided in their countries. In several countries (Australia, Canada, Ireland, Italy, Japan, Spain, South Korea, and the United Kingdom), nurse scholars have developed conceptualizations that are specifically derived from the history and culture of nursing in their country. In several other countries (Egypt, Israel, Jordan, Mexico, and Thailand), the nurse scholars have adapted conceptualizations from theories developed by scholars from the United States. In these latter chapters the authors describe the relevance to the theories to nursing in their own country and culture, and provide examples of how the theories have been applied to research and professional practice.

WHY WE DID THIS BOOK?

We are proud to be scholars nursing and are committed to advancing the profession through both theoretical development and applications of theories to research and professional practice. We initiated this book project because we believed that the stories of theoretical developments from our global colleagues in nursing would help future nurse scholars everywhere in their quest for scientific excellence. Throughout the world professional nurses make a difference in the lives of those they serve, with intentional directed compassionate care. We believe that the science development must be as deliberate as the professional practice development.

We initiated this book to expand our knowledge of what nurse theorists in other countries are thinking and doing, and to engage our nursing theory colleagues in sharing their theoretical understandings embedded in their country and culture. We are indebted to the chapter authors for their contributions and for their persistence in expanding understandings of the work we do as nurse scholars, researchers, and clinicians. Throughout the last several years, we have been very cognizant of the continued need for theory development in nursing globally. It is in the profound spirit of expanding knowledge development for the nursing discipline that led us to invite global colleagues to share their understandings of the discipline. This book represents an investment in the future of global nursing.

Joyce J. Fitzpatrick

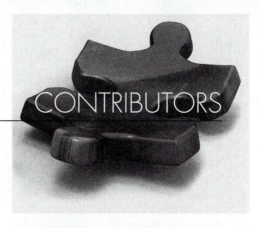

CONTRIBUTORS

Muayyad M. Ahmad, PhD, RN
Professor
Clinical Nursing Department
The University of Jordan
Amman, Jordan

Merav Ben-Natan, PhD, RN
Director
Hillel-Yaffe Academic School of Nursing
Hadera, Isreal

Montserrat Valverde Bosch, MNS, RN
Director of Nursing at the Haemato-
Oncology Institute
Hospital Clínic of Barcelona
Barcelona, Spain

Roser Cadena, MSc, RN
Assistant Director of Nursing
Hospital Clínic of Barcelona
Barcelona, Spain

Emili Comas, RN, CNS
Director of Nursing
Gynecology, Obstetrics and Neonatology
Institute
Hospital Clinic of Barcelona
Barcelona, Spain

Latefa A. Dardas, MSc, RN
Community Health Nursing Deptartment
The University of Jordan
Amman, Jordan

Mally Ehrenfeld, PhD, RN
Associate Professor
Department of Nursing
School of Health Professions
Tel Aviv University
Tel Aviv, Israel

Joyce J. Fitzpatrick, PhD, MBA, RN, FAAN, FNAP
Elizabeth Brooks Ford Professor
of Nursing
Frances Payne Bolton School
of Nursing
Case Western Reserve
University
Cleveland, Ohio

M. Teresa Fusté, MN, RN, CNS
Director of Nursing at the Neurosciences
Institute
Hospital Clínic of Barcelona
Barcelona, Spain

Esther C. Gallegos PhD, RN
Profesor Titular "B"
Facultad de Enfermería
Universidad Autonoma de
Nuevo Leon
Monterrey, Mexico

Margaret M. Glembocki, DNP, RN, ACNP-BC, CSC, FAANP
Assistant Professor
School of Nursing
Oakland University
Rochester, Michigan

Laurie N. Gottlieb, PhD, RN
Professor
Flora Madeline Shaw Chair
of Nursing
Ingram School of Nursing
McGill University
Nurse Scholar-in-Residence
Jewish General Hospital
Montreal, QC, Canada

Michal Itzhaki, PhD, RN
Lecturer
Nursing Department
School of Health Professions
Tel Aviv University
Tel Aviv, Israel

Younhee Kang, PhD, RN, ANP
Professor
College of Health Sciences
Ewha Womans University,
Seoul, South Korea

Susie Kim, DNSc, RN, FAAN
Principle and Professor
Daeyang College of Nursing
Lilongwe, Malawi

**Margaret Landers, PhD, MSc,
RGN, RM**
College Lecturer
Catherine McAuley School of Nursing
and Midwifery
University College
Cork, Ireland

Haeok Lee, PhD, RN, FAAN
Professor
College of Nursing and Health Sciences
University of Massachusetts
Boston, Massachusetts

**Tanya McCance, DPhil, MSc,
BSc, RGN**
Head
Person-Centered Practice Research Centre
Institute of Nursing and Health Research
Faculty of Life and Health Sciences
University of Ulster
Ulster, Northern Ireland

**Geraldine McCarthy, PhD, MSN,
MEd, RGN**
Emerita Professor
Catherine McAuley School of Nursing
and Midwifery
University College Cork
Cork, Ireland

**Brendan McCormack, D.Phil, BSC,
FRCN, PGCEA, RGN, RMN, FEANS**
Head of the Division of Nursing,
Queen Margaret University
Edinburgh, Scotland

Rungnapa Panitrat, PhD, RN
Department of Mental Health
and Psychiatric Nursing
Faculty of Nursing
Mahidol University
Bangkok, Thailand

Wanpen Piyopasakul, PhD, RN
Department of Medical Nursing
Faculty of Nursing
Mahidol University
Bangkok, Thailand

Norma Ponzoni, MScN, MEd, RN
Faculty Lecturer
Ingram School of Nursing
McGill University
Montreal, QC, Canada

**Bertha Cecilia Salazar-González, PhD,
MA, RN**
Profesor Titular "B"
College of Nursing
Universidad Autonoma de Nuevo Leon
Monterrey, Mexico

Pedro Sanz, MN, RN
Director of Nursing at the Diagnostic
Imaging Center
Hospital Clínic of Barcelona
Barcelona, Spain

Mary Jane Smith, PhD, RN
Professor of Nursing
West Virginia University
Morgantown, West Virginia

Natawon Suwonnaroop, PhD, RN
Department of Public Health
Nursing
Faculty of Nursing
Mahidol University
Bangkok, Thailand

Ann L. Whall, PhD, RN FAAN
Maggie Allesee Endowed Professor
Geriatric Nursing Research
School of Nursing
Oakland University
Rochester, MI
Professor Emerita
University of Michigan
Ann Arbor, Michigan

Jill White, PhD, RN, RM
Professor
Faculty of Nursing and Midwifery
University of Sydney
Camperdown, NSW, Australia

Toyoaki Yamauchi, MD, ND, PhD
Graduate School of Medicine,
Department of Nursing,
Nagoya University
Nagoya, Japan

Adelaida Zabalegui, PhD, RN, FEANS
Chief Executive Officer of Nursing
Hospital Clínic of Barcelona
Barcelona, Spain

Renzo Zanotti, PhD, RN, FEANS
Associate Professor of Nursing
Dean of Nursing
School of Medicine and Surgery
University of Padova
Padova, Italy

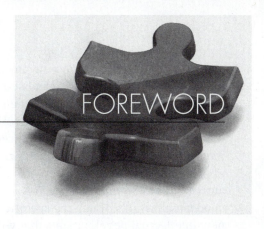

FOREWORD

Mary Jane Smith

This text will be particularly appealing to students, faculty, and nurse administrators who are interested in expanding their worldview about the current state of nursing theory from a global perspective. This perspective opens one's understanding of nursing knowledge in greater depth and breadth. Depth comes with understanding the view of the metaparadigm described in each chapter, and breadth comes from the perspective of specific frameworks that can be found in each. Thus, the authors provide a perspective of how nursing is conceptualized in other countries and give voice to a community of scholars that extends beyond the borders of the United States.

The chapters in this text have been written by individuals who have taken responsibility for advancing nursing conceptual models in their country. Thirteen countries are represented. Eight authors have described unique models, and five have described the application of existing models that were developed in the United States. Models presented in the text represent a movement to think about nursing conceptually, away from a narrow point of view to a holistic one. Several holistic models described in the text are strength-based nursing, personhood, health as harmony, and interpersonal caring. Along with the holistic view, the concept of culture shines through in many of the models. Several cultural viewpoints presented are Aboriginal and Torres Strait Islander, Russian Israeli, Arab Muslim, and Irish Catholic. Several chapter authors identify the importance of focusing on culture as a major influence on the understandings that guide nurses both in knowledge development and professional practice. This point is worth highlighting as a contribution to nursing scholarship. The health of individuals cannot be separated from the cultures in which they live. These cultural understandings are relevant with the increased diversity throughout the world.

As the world grows more connected, a push for knowledge from an international perspective is mandated. In this shared space of knowledge development is a growing interdependence that has advanced with rapid telecommunications and ease of travel across the world. The space is occupied by gatherings at international meetings and at nursing programs where international students come together. The chapters in this text provide an opportunity for discussion, debate, and dialogue in this shared space. The authors are to be commended for accepting the challenge of articulating conceptualizations of nursing specific to their countries. Some of these are new intellectual developments that will spur further intellectual discourse and applications in science development. Each of these conceptualizations challenges nurses everywhere to think deeply about the foundations of nursing knowledge and the need for continued application in education, research, and professional nursing practice.

Mary Jane Smith, PhD, RN
Professor of Nursing
West Virginia University
Morgantown, West Virginia

CONCEPTUAL MODELS OF NURSING

Global Perspectives

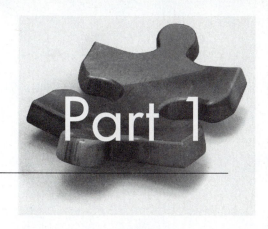

Part 1

Foundations for the Globalization of Nursing

CHAPTER OUTLINE

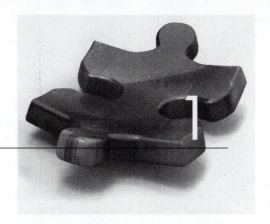

Nursing Knowledge Development: Mandate for a Global Nursing Perspective

Joyce J. Fitzpatrick

Never before has the global imperative for the nursing discipline been so striking. The more than 16 million nurses face global challenges and opportunities, not only to make a difference in further defining the disciplinary perspective of nursing but also to contribute to solving global health challenges.

Yet, nursing remains an evolving discipline, both in its science development (theory and research) and its professional practice. As nurses we trace our disciplinary perspectives in modern nursing to the work of Florence Nightingale who shaped not only the way we think about our educational preparation, but also the work that we do to enhance quality and safety, to influence public and institutional policy, and to generate and communicate the scientific rationale for our direct care provided to patients, families, and communities.

Today, our science includes the integration of grand theories with practice-level theory. More recently, there has been an emphasis on building middle-range theory to guide both our science and professional practice.

Nursing conceptual models are understood to include nursing philosophies, disciplinary beliefs, understandings, and purposes. Flowing from these grand theories are the middle-range and practice theories that are more closely associated both conceptually and practically to the everyday activities of nurse educators, researchers, and clinicians. This deductive

3

process of theory development leads nurses to discover new ideals and potential applications of knowledge. Yet scientists also can engage in inductive processes of building knowledge from their observations of data, both clinical data and understanding as well as discrete scientific data. Both processes have great relevance for the discipline of nursing.

Nursing conceptual models also provide the overall direction for nursing practice, education, and research. Components of basic and applied research, ethics, and knowledge from philosophical and historical inquiry can be derived from these broad conceptualizations. The research and professional practice of the discipline also include integration of knowledge from other disciplines, particularly the health sciences. Several examples of the integration of disciplinary knowledge and reformulation according to the nursing conceptualization can be found in the recent book by Fitzpatrick and McCarthy (2014). The authors delineate new understandings of theories originally developed within disciplines such as psychology and sociology. The relevance of these theories to nursing research and professional practice are made explicit as are conceptualizations from several grand- and middle-range theories in nursing.

Although it is imperative to address the process of our knowledge development in nursing, its content is also critical. Both process and content components of the knowledge within the nursing discipline are embedded in nursing conceptual models and the middle-range and practice theories that flow from these models or serve as the foundation to build the conceptual models.

This chapter addresses the following questions: What is science? What is the nature of knowing in a science and a professional practice? How do the patterns of knowing of the scientist and professional practitioner complement each other?

Science represents one means of understanding ourselves and our world. Disciplines develop when there is a convergence of thought across dominant groups within the disciplines. Yet these disciplinary perspectives must be communicated to the rank-and-file scientists and practitioners in order for there to be acceptance and further discourse and refinement. We are at an early stage of nursing knowledge development within global nursing scientific circles. This stage is focused on making the knowledge more explicit across geographic boundaries. Once we understand the commonalities within our global scientific perspectives, we can move forward to further develop and refine our science and professional practice, remaining cognizant of the need to respect cultural differences that will continue to shape the specific disciplinary perspectives.

In a clinical discipline such as nursing, there are two distinct ways of knowing, requiring different skill sets (Fitzpatrick, 2002, 2003). One way comes from clinicians, particularly those who are experts, who develop knowledge through a process of synthesizing information quickly. They make clinical judgments based on the rapid synthesis of information. The more expert the clinician, the more quickly the information can be synthesized, and the more accurate the clinical judgment will be. Clinical scholars use knowledge developed through evidence-based practice to further advance their clinical understandings. Best practices inform current clinical practice, and the clinical scholar relies on evidence from a variety of sources to guide clinical judgment.

In addition to clinical knowledge development through expert clinical practice, we also develop nursing knowledge through use of the scientific process, including theory development and research. Researchers view the world by examining each component in great depth. They are much more likely to proceed cautiously, viewing each detail from many different perspectives and gathering much data before reaching conclusions. The research process takes things apart, and only after considerable data collection and analyses does the researcher arrive at interpretations and conclusions.

It is not common for the expert researcher to also be an expert clinician. Rather, because a different skill set is required of each, the most effective teams for developing knowledge within a clinical discipline such as nursing would include both expert clinicians and expert scientists. Each partner would bring his or her different skill set to the knowledge development process.

Both research and clinical practice are guided by general and specific understandings of the world. At times, the broad understandings are referred to as "world views." As these views have become more deliberate and more systematically developed within the nursing discipline, they have been understood as nursing conceptual models. As models and frameworks, these structures provide the foundation for the development of both clinical and scientific knowledge. These models provide both the form (structures) and the content that are the base for nursing science and professional practice. The more specific understandings are referred to as *theories*. Both the broad conceptualizations and the specific theories guide us in the development of science and professional practice.

Nursing as a discipline must attend to both the process of knowledge development and the content of nursing knowledge, particularly as we move into the global arena. The nurse scientist and the nurse clinician must have the tools with which to develop their knowledge. Multiple modes of inquiry within both research and clinical practice are warranted, especially because nursing has staked a knowledge claim to understanding holistic persons and their health. Nurse scientists and clinicians together can develop knowledge that builds the holistic framework, thus adding a dimension of knowledge that is not developed through other disciplines or through the application of knowledge from these other disciplines to professional nursing practice. This is particularly important as we expand our knowledge boundaries within nursing to encompass nursing disciplinary content throughout the globe.

Quality research is rather simple to identify from a general scientific standard. Peer-reviewed evaluation of the merit of research serves as the basic criterion, including the use of the peer review process in judging both the award of research funds and the acceptance of research manuscripts in scientific journals. Quality theory is also possible to evaluate, although a different set of criteria is used. There exists a basic set of evaluation criteria that is consistent across levels of theory. There also exists a set of standards upon which clinical knowledge can be judged. Thus, each component of knowledge development has its own parameters for judging the quality of the work.

Some characteristics are desirable in both clinical scholarship and science development. Knowledge development from wider approach would be enhanced by attention to the desired outcomes and anticipated products of the knowledge development processes whether developed through clinical scholarship or research. Outcome-driven models are most valued in contemporary professional work. Thus, both the clinical and the scientific ways of knowing in nursing should be built on strong foundations of inquiry with attention to process, content, and outcome of the inquiry.

Clinical and scientific scholarship is likely to flourish in environments where there is support for knowledge development, including attention to nurturing innovation and creativity. Attention to the outcomes of knowledge development is a very important factor. Improvements in clinical outcomes now serve as important criteria by which we judge our clinical interventions and our overall clinical practice. This is true throughout the globe in nursing and health care. The use of clinical knowledge is also important in anticipating and predicting needs for health care services as well as designing and managing these services once the needs are identified. As clinical scholars become more experienced, it is important for them to assume an active role in creating the environments in which knowledge development can advance. In addition, as scientists become more attuned to the clinical phenomena uncovered by partners in professional nursing practice, they can engage in scholarship that is directly relevant to health outcomes of the individuals, families, and communities they serve.

In summary, it can best be understood that clinical scholarship and research together provide the core knowledge on which expert professional nursing practice is developed, locally and globally. Both the clinical and scientific knowledge are essential to inform a clinical discipline such as nursing; they are intertwined and interdependent. Both benefit from the strengths inherent in a knowledge development approach that incorporates attention to these interrelated ways of knowing. Furthermore, our global nursing knowledge will be enhanced by sharing details of both clinical and scientific knowledge development.

REFERENCES

Fitzpatrick, J. J. (2002). The balance in nursing: Clinical and scientific ways of knowing and being. *Nursing Education Perspectives, 23,* 57.

Fitzpatrick, J. J. (2003). The case for the clinical doctorate. *Reflections in Nursing Leadership, 29,* 8, 9, 13.

Fitzpatrick, J. J., & McCarthy, G. (Eds.). (2014). *Theories guiding nursing research and practice.* New York: Springer.

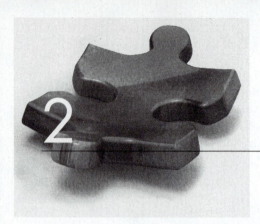

2

Philosophy of Science Positions and Their Importance in Cross-National Nursing

Ann L. Whall

INTRODUCTION

Positions regarding several tenets of scientific philosophy have challenged as well as supported the idea that nursing is an individual and increasingly important science, worthy of acceptance and taught in a school or college in major universities, not only in the United States but also worldwide. A cursory review of important U.S. nursing journals and texts supports the relevance of cross-national discussions to this position (Almutairi & Rondney, 2013; Baird, 2012; Hunter, et al., 2013; Tasci-Duran & Sevil, 2013; McCarthy & Fitzpatrick, 2012). These journals, texts, and other equally significant U.S. nursing sources, have identified "global nursing" sections, thus supporting the importance of cross-national discussions on substantive issues discussed here. No subject is likely of more importance to cross-national discussions than that of the philosophic base of nursing's theoretic body of knowledge.

This discussion begins by defining these terms: *Theory* is defined in a structural manner, that is, as a group of concepts, interrelated via propositional statements, that is based on a group of underlying assumptions. Likewise, the *philosophy of science* is defined as the examination of disciplinary elements from a philosophic perspective. The term *discipline of nursing* is defined in the Donaldson and Crowley (1977) manner (i.e., as including all aspects and levels of nursing science, education, and practice). These disciplinary elements form the knowledge base of nursing, which (as characterized by Carper, 1978) are nursing's keys to knowledge. Carper's four "ways of knowing" are briefly referred to here as scientific, artistic/ aesthetic, experiential, and ethical. They display different philosophies of science positions that are described later. In cross-national nursing discussions, positions of the philosophy of science are considered important but have some confusing areas.

One of the clearest discussions of the ways in which different positions regarding the philosophy of science directly affect the development of an integrated body of disciplinary knowledge is found in the discipline of astrophysics. One position of the philosophy of science was the subject of disagreement between Einstein's causal view and the proponents of quantum mechanics who took an opposite or probabilistic view. Einstein's oft quoted comment characterizes this disagreement, "God does not play dice" (i.e., foundational astrophysics relationships are causal, not probabilistic in nature). The competition between these two philosophies of science are cross-national in nature. In Greene's view, this competition slowed scientific progress in astrophysics. Discussion of these differences and how they have been addressed well in nursing helps to prevent cross-national misunderstanding.

Related Discussions in Nursing

Beginning about mid-20th century and when philosophic discussions in astrophysics were taking place, many Ph.D. programs in nursing were offered in the United States. These discussions concerned a "causal" position of philosophy of science known as *logical positivism* (LP), which many people saw as the primary and basic philosophy of science underlying *all* science, including the discipline of nursing. Consequently, if nursing were judged by the LP position alone, it was often seen as unscientific in nature and thus unfit for university status.

Analytic discussions concerning the nursing discipline in the United States demonstrated, however, that although certain aspects of nursing knowledge (i.e., "scientific ways of knowing"; see Carper's analysis) might be evaluated appropriately using LP causal criteria, Carper's other ways of knowing (i.e., the ethical, aesthetic, personal/experiential, ways of knowing; Whall, 1986) would not and should not be judged by that position alone. There is another reason that an LP causal position alone is inadequate to judge "nursing's scientific way of knowing" because all nursing has at least three levels of theoretical knowledge or theory. They are the (1) grand or conceptual model level that contains abstract generalized theory with extremely broad or summative concepts, (2) the middle range or less abstract and, thus, a more measurable level with specific concepts, and (3) the specific and/or measurable microlevel practice theories. Once these levels of theory were generally understood and accepted, the application of criteria to all three levels of nursing knowledge was seen as inappropriate. This led nursing in United States to apply a more probabilistic philosophy of science often known as *neomodernism* (discussed subsequently) to nursing knowledge.

In summary, the argument in astrophysics regarding the requirement that its body of knowledge must consider relationships/propositions as being causal rather than probabilistic in nature also was applied to nursing in the United States. After initial rather caustic evaluations of the body of nursing knowledge as being inadequate and nonscientific from an LP perspective, this perspective was revised; nursing knowledge was assessed in essence to be composed of other important types of knowledge that were not only causal but also aesthetic-artistic, ethical, and experiential in nature. These other ways of knowing reflected more of the probabilistic approach known as *neomodernism*. This newer, broader neomodern approach led to a clearer acceptance of the body of nursing knowledge in universities and the discipline of nursing itself.

Furthermore, in the United States, the ongoing analysis and evaluation of the conceptual models or grand theory of nursing led to increasing recognition that at all three levels (grand, middle range, and micro) of nursing theory should more appropriately be evaluated in the following ways: Causal relationships aspired to in an LP approach would be more appropriate for analyzing and evaluating nursing's microlevel practice theory and, to a lower extent, the middle range level, but the grand theories are more appropriately judged via probabilistic criteria.

Recurring Issues in the Discussion of Nursing Theory in the United States

Although it might seem that in the United States the much sought-after integrated body of nursing knowledge, having been well defined and defended, is now well understood and accepted, this is not always the case. Periodically, a harkening back to simpler times is called for with a plea for the nursing discipline to include only the LP causal, "hands-on" practice approach as nursing knowledge. Among the reason is perhaps that "just sticking to practice" seems simpler and less esoteric than seeking to develop an integrated overall body of nursing knowledge. Thus in 1993 and 2004, several suggestions were made to discard more abstract theoretic issues and discussions of nursing and to produce "just practical" knowledge. Of course, practical nursing programs usually of one year were available outside universities, but this was not the prevailing attitude. In 2004 when the important DNP (doctorate in nursing practice) programs were initially being discussed, a similar suggestion was made, but this time the plea was to eliminate all metatheoretical discussions from DNP programs (Whall, 2005).

Unfortunately, the reality is that unless the greatly needed DNP practitioners understand the philosophic bases for nursing, they can mimic philosophies of other disciplines that do not reflect nursing's four ways of knowing and revert to a more causal approach to their practice. A nonphilosophic-based practice in nursing leads to aberrant nursing attitudes and practices (e.g., Nurse Ratched's approach in the film *One Flew over the Cuckoo's Nest*). Therefore, understanding nursing's foundational philosophic position and the four ways of knowing is essential. Such issues, although metatheoretical in nature, will define and control the nature of the DNP nursing practice area.

Kim (2011, xi) summarized the preceding discussion regarding the need to understand metatheoretical issues in both basic and advanced nursing:

> Nursing's knowledge system as a human practice science is concerned with developing knowledge for practice; the knowledge that is relevant to and needed in practice. As a human practice science, nursing has to address epistemic questions regarding specific human conditions within the nursing domains and those related to how to improve such human conditions from the nursing perspective. . . . Unfortunately, the development of nursing knowledge during the past several decades has followed the course that has been mapped out and followed by various scientific fields within which the objectification of subject matters is the primary mode of scientific work.

Developing an Integrated Body of Nursing Knowledge

This discussion is based on the assumption that each nation has in its history a set of beliefs and understandings regarding the origin, nature, and development of its own discipline of nursing. It is further understood that the steps discussed here are primarily U.S. or at least western in nature and that every step addressing development of an integrated body of nursing knowledge cannot be appropriate to every nation. However, the steps described later compose one approach offered as a possible means by which other nations and countries might seek to further develop the body of their nursing knowledge. Furthermore, these steps are presented as discrete and separate—which in reality is not the case—because they are ongoing and integrated in nature.

PHILOSOPHIC ISSUES

We begin this theoretical explication by focusing on philosophic issues and defining the philosophy of science positions that are characteristic to nursing in the United States. Because it is likely that there are similarities in the nursing discipline across nations, a preliminary analysis procedure developed cross-nationally is needed to clarify each nation's methods.

Philosophic Analysis as Method

The philosophic analysis steps developed and applied by Whall and Hicks are to (a) identify selected themes in a given area of interest, (b) examine the discussions concerning these themes from three philosophic positions (discussed next) to identify types of agreement and/or disagreement, (c) identify and use *metanarratives* (defined as overarching disciplinary beliefs) extracted from discussions of these themes, and (d) develop exemplar cases to further explicate the issues. In the Whall and Hicks discussion, the topic of interest was evidence-based nursing; these four steps were used in a philosophic analysis of several issues in a given nation's discipline to clarify cross-national practices.

Because it is likely that the philosophy of science positions affecting nursing in other nations differ from the U.S. position, an overview of the three most relevant philosophic positions regarding the discipline of nursing—positivism, postmodernism, and neomodernism—are discussed next.

Positivism

Positivism, one variation of which was logical positivism, dominated scientific thought beginning in the mid-19th century (Whall & Hicks, 2002). One variation of logical positivism's major tenets, the verification principle, had great impact on both nursing theory and research; it posited that phenomena were scientifically meaningful only if they were empirically verifiable via sense experience and/or logical proof (Phillips, 1987). Although the empirics in nursing can take many forms (and generally do not reflect a strict verification perspective), the influence of positivism affects segments of nursing practice, education, and research (Whall, 1989). Positivism supports a "context-stripping" approach in which various aspects of situations—especially contextual aspects that cannot be directly operationalized—are seen as unimportant. This viewpoint is contrary to nursing's historic perspective, which has dealt with patient values and meanings (e.g., spiritual desires and cultural beliefs) that arguably affect virtually all nursing situations. Many in nursing saw the verificationist perspective of positivism as being greatly restrictive and, therefore was not fully or generally embraced in nursing education and practice.

Postmodernism

Postmodern thinking was in large part a reaction to the restrictive views of science of positivism but also was a result of multiple other societal and philosophical influences. Postmodernism made its appearance in scientific discussions sometime around the beginning of the 20th century, although it was not recognized or seen as influential in nursing in the United States until approximately the last decade of the 20th century (Whall & Hicks, 2002).

Postmodernists criticized the universal claims of the positivists regarding scientific truth (Abbey, 2000; Schrag, 1997). Postmodernists characterized positivists as "context strippers," denoting inattention to the reciprocal relationships between individuals and their many environments and objectifying those that were observed. Nursing cannot ignore the context of persons, however, because clinical situations are often chaotic and characterized by multiple, diverse, and simultaneous interactions that are virtually uncontrollable.

Many characteristics of postmodernism are congruent with traditional nursing values and experiences. Likewise, nursing theorists for the most part deviated in both educational background and research training from that of scientists holding strict positivist views. When the postmodernist movement expanded the possibilities for science, newly accepted topics for theory and research afforded the discipline both interesting and fuller possibilities not available in a positivistic world. A great criticism of postmodernism, however, is the tendency to overanalyze, overevaluate, deconstruct, and provide few alternatives for reconstruction via the synthesis of such findings. This position has led some in nursing and other disciplines to accept all viewpoints as having equal merit, leading to much confusion.

Multiple conceptual nursing models were developed during an era of great postmodern influence; the models reflect postmodern views and sometimes certain positivistic views. The focus here is on both analysis and evaluation of three levels of nursing theory—grand or conceptual, middle range, and microlevel practice—and on the synthesis of these outcomes for nursing practice; such an effort might be seen as most reflective of a neomodernist position.

Neomodernism

External to nursing (and often European in origin), a shift in the scientific worldview (from positivism to postmodernism and then to neomodernism) has been a major topic of discussion for several years. The discussions by Laudan (1977) and Lakatos (1977) view science in a newer manner (Whall & Hicks, 2002). Laudan saw science as progressing and guided by a collection of assumptions, tools, methods, axioms, and principles. Many theories could reside in this view, but some commonalities grounded in the past sometimes remained. Laudan's views are now more descriptive of the state of the discipline of nursing. Reed (1995) and others use the term *neomodernism* to describe the state of science that goes beyond both positivism and post-modernism. This "above-and-beyond" characteristic of neomodernism is an approach to science in which a deliberative effort is made to use important traditional metanarratives (such as those found in grand theories and conceptual nursing models) to address current problems in science.

In Reed's view, the neomodernist approach includes the freedom to explore and propose alternative methods to be included in nursing science while considering important historic values and traditions. Neomodernism, therefore, offers a more inclusive and seemingly more liberated perspective than even postmodernism and suggests an important role for conceptual nursing models as excellent sources of nursing metanarratives in this "new" science. *Metanarratives* in neomodernism are defined as important enduring themes found in disciplinary products such as the conceptual nursing models.

Other Philosophic Issues

Philosophy in large part concerns what are termed *ontological* and *epistemological questions. Ontology* is a branch of philosophy addressing the nature of reality (Reed, 1997; Arslanian-Engoren, 2005). Theory in a discipline is influenced by ontological assumptions about what exists and how we know what we know. Ontology, for example, can deal with the questions of reality.

Ontological issues in nursing have been addressed many times. For example, during the 1960s, nursing assumed the validity of a then-popular theory that schizophrenia was caused by cold and rejecting mothers. Later, however, when it was possible to visualize brain function, nursing came to accept that schizophrenia most likely existed because of impaired neurologic mechanisms. Data incongruent with the theory of the schizophrenic mother were then used to modify the understanding of schizophrenia and how nursing might work with persons afflicted with it and their families.

The discussion of the ways of knowing in nursing is of an epistemological nature (Carper, 1978); *epistemology* in this sense concerns the structure of knowledge. The value of issues such as nursing diagnoses, Nursing Interventions Classification (NICs), and Nursing Outcomes Classification (NOCs) systems in the discipline have been debated. Likewise, whether nursing theory could or should be deductively structured from nursing grand theories, inductively derived from practice, or both have been discussions of an epistemological nature. Therefore, discussions in nursing about the value of disciplinary products, especially in cross-national nursing discussions, are epistemological in nature and based on the philosophic positions in nursing in a given country.

The neomodernist position currently influencing nursing considers many conflicting viewpoints to be useful. Such views include the recognition that nurse practitioners need to remain aware of multiple understandings of various phenomena and that this knowledge could restructure their practice. Neomodernism finds that the usefulness of such scholarly products of the discipline, such as research findings, could and would be guided by nursing metanarratives (or nursing's historic beliefs and themes). It is thus essential that this neomodernist position be examined closely and its influence on cross-national nursing be understood.

The neomodernist position posits that reality is likely or potentially flawed and that examining multiple ways of knowing is one way to attempt to establish an acceptable "reality" for nursing (for a time). Discussions in and across nations about the nature of certain topics such as evidence-based practice (EBP) are, therefore, important. For example, the nature of the role that experiential knowledge plays in EBP is an important issue (Whall, Sinclair, & Paraboo, 2006).

PERSPECTIVE, DOMAINS, PERSISTENT QUESTIONS, AND TRUTH CRITERIA IN NURSING IN THE UNITED STATES

Ellis was a clear-thinking, futuristic scholar who concerned herself with major questions regarding the structure of nursing knowledge. The editors of this text, as members of a nursing theory think tank, noted Ellis' belief that by addressing structural questions first, one might better understand current nursing issues in the United States. Nursing science, according to Ellis, is composed of both processes and products; thus, debate (e.g., a scientific process) about nursing products (e.g., nursing models) is needed in the United States. Both of these scientific elements (products and processes) are important in a neomodernist view of nursing.

According to Ellis, the major components of the structure of the nursing discipline are *perspective, domains, persistent questions, truth criteria,* and *the community of scholars* (Algase & Whall, 1993, 1995). There are other elements, such as those outlined by Phoenix (1964), but Ellis often focused on these five components.

The *domains* of the discipline are the subjects or content areas on which nursing practice focuses. One might conceptualize this content using older terms (e.g., medical surgical nursing or pediatrics) or using more contemporary terms (e.g., long-term care, critical care). According to Algase & Whall (1993), it is important to realize that no one discipline "owns" any particular area of knowledge; in the marketplace of ideas, a given discipline can claim any area or at least address that area in its own disciplinary manner. Knowledge across disciplines is gradually modified and then becomes accepted in other disciplines. For example, monitoring blood pressure and using electrocardiography in the United States were at first part of medical knowledge and later became part of nursing practice. Nursing focuses on caregiving as do other disciplines such as social work. Thus, the domains or components of knowledge found in any one discipline have a history, fluctuate, can be shared with other disciplines, and can be relatively identified only as specific to a particular discipline at a point in time.

The *perspective* of a discipline is perhaps the most fascinating structural element that Ellis discussed, for it is composed in large part of historical and traditional precedents, philosophical and ethical components, visionary ideals, and commonly accepted practices. This perspective of nursing in any nation is important because it can be used to identify and sanction what can be considered "nursing" theory, "nursing" research, and "nursing" practice. In other words, the way in which given domains of a science are addressed (and their distinction from other disciplines) is largely the result of perspective.

Perspective is also used to evaluate the content of the domains. An example of this evaluative function is the debate over advanced-practice knowledge in nursing. Once the preserve or domain of physicians alone, in-depth physical assessment knowledge has gradually become part of the primary assessment of advanced-practice nursing. A debate in nursing between traditionalists and nontraditionalists has stimulated opposing views with regard to such assessment. One group (the traditionalists) sees in-depth physical assessment as a normal extension of the domain of nursing, believing that as technology advances, domains are modified. This "avant-garde" (nontraditionalist) group argues that although this assessment procedure is used in many disciplines, the perspective of a given discipline determines how and why it is applied. The perspectives of all disciplines are somewhat and relatively in a state of flux but also contain stable elements, such as identifiable metanarratives across time.

The *persistent questions* in the nursing discipline in the United States apply to the discipline's practice, education, and research discussions and clearly involve the products of nursing science: "Was the action ethical?" and "Was the holistic perspective of nursing evident?" are examples of such questions. They also currently address trends in nursing research in the United States over time; questions regarding cost-benefit analysis provide one such example.

The *truth criteria* used in the United States to evaluate nursing products are traditional as well as evolving. The analysis and evaluation guidelines used in this text in essence compose one type of truth criteria. Questions used by national accrediting bodies, state boards, institutional review boards, and human subject review groups also represent nursing's institutionalized truth criteria.

The *community of scholars* across nations is composed of members of the nursing discipline who seek to develop it by broadening the knowledge base of nursing through activities such as research, scholarly discussions, and debates. The community of scholars, in Ellis' view, should be involved in questions that address issues at the "cutting edge" of the nursing discipline worldwide.

Ellis in essence believed one threat to the community of scholars was that its "scholarly" pursuits and debates might become so esoteric that they would become estranged from nursing practice and nursing practitioners. For example, most practicing nurses did not know about the debate regarding logical positivism (Whall, 1989) and never considered rejecting the spiritual aspect of care as "unscientific." Nursing scholars, therefore, must continually check the relevance of their scholarly pursuits and debates; at times, they lead the discipline and at times, they follow it, but in Ellis' view, these scholars need to maintain their relevancy to nursing practice.

ANALYSIS AND EVALUATION OF THREE LEVELS OF NURSING THEORY OR KNOWLEDGE

Important to any discipline is knowledge of the status of its accepted theories. Status is determined by ongoing analyses of the theoretic base. Nursing in the United States has a long history of developing the correct criteria with which to evaluate the discipline's theoretical base. The following discussion of the manner in which nursing's theoretical base has been validly and reliably evaluated is derived from and based on nursing's truth criteria and from conceptual nursing models and other early metatheoretical discussion in nursing.

The analysis and evaluation criteria used for the three model levels of nursing theory (micropractice, middle range, and grand or conceptual) have been modified to be relevant to the characteristics of each level. It is also important to keep in mind that the assumptions at each level differ in causality and probability that likely vary across nations. As discussed previously, grand-level theories (e.g., conceptual nursing models) contain abstract concepts regarding persons, their environment, and health that are summative in nature because each refers to all persons, all environments, and all health as well as all of nursing. The propositional statements in this level of theory are for the most part probabilistic in nature rather than causal.

Practice or Microtheory

Practice-level theory, also called *microtheory* and *prescriptive theory,* is more specific or concrete than the other two levels of theory and addresses specific directions and prescriptions for practice. Research on decubitus ulcers, nasal gastric suction, and urinary catheterization, for example, can be readily identified as practice-level theory. It is also the product of other methods including induction from practice, deduction from middle-range theory (MRT), and research on conceptual nursing models. Many of nursing's early guidelines for care, which are found in hospital procedure books, describe practice theory generated inductively and primarily from practical experience using trial-and-error methods. In this level of theory, causal statements are common; for example, hand washing for a certain amount of time and in a particular way eliminates pathogens on the hands.

The work of Benner, Hooper-Kytiakidis, & Stannard (1999) addresses an interesting manner in which expert practice knowledge can be chronicled. They describe an interpretive process in which nurses keep records of exemplar cases concerning clinical patterns. By (in part) reflecting on these narratives, nurses can produce practice-level knowledge, which suggests a "thinking-in-action" approach to practice-level theory and knowledge development. This thinking in action is based, however, on an in-depth understanding of the situation as opposed to strictly a rule-bound approach.

The work of Johnson and Ratner (1997) suggests a similar developmental process for practice-level theory or knowledge. They support the idea that one can "theorize" about practical application knowledge and/or capture it in theory and that this "thinking-in-action" is an ongoing process. As discussed earlier, this microlevel theory is likely to have more causal propositional statements that refer to specific or nonsummative objects and situations. Therefore, causal statements are appropriate in practice theory because the microlevel concepts can be directly observed and manipulated.

This is in opposition to summative concepts, which cannot be directly observed (e.g., observing all of humanity in one instance), nor can they be directly manipulated.

The guidelines for analysis and evaluation of nursing practice theory in the United States are in the form of questions that will lead to practice actions. These guidelines do not address the analysis of the four metaparadigm concepts of person, environment, health, and nursing (as used for evaluation of conceptual nursing models); instead, these concepts are seen as implicit to the questions. Because practice theory is designed for immediate application to practice, questions regarding the match or fit with existing empirical data are most important. Likewise, the relevance and adequacy for immediate application to practice of concept definitions are important. Operational definitions, which describe how to apply practice theory, are important for practice theory. Thus, the adequacy of operational definitions is addressed.

It is important to note again that the following criteria have been developed in the context of nursing discussions and applications in the United States. Therefore, each nation using these steps to evaluate its theory must discuss and apply them in the context of that country's specific disciplinary knowledge.

TABLE 2–1   Criteria for the Cross-National Analysis and Evaluation of Practice Theory in a Given Nation

Basic Considerations
1. Definitional adequacy: Can the concepts be readily operationalized?
2. Empirical adequacy: Are the operationalized concepts congruent with empirical data?
3. Statement/propositional adequacy: Do the statements lead to clear directives for nursing care? Are the statements sufficient to the practice task at hand and are not contradictory in nature?

Internal Analysis and Evaluation
1. Consideration of completeness and consistency: Are there gaps or inconsistencies in the theory that could lead to prescriptive conflicts and difficulties?
2. Assumptions of theory: Are these beliefs congruent with nursing's historical perspective? Are these assumptions congruent with existing ethical standards and social policy? Do these assumptions conflict with those of given cultural groups?

External Analysis and Evaluation
1. Analysis of existing standards: Is the practice theory produced congruent with existing nursing standards? Is the practice theory produced congruent with care standards produced external to nursing (e.g., by the Agency for Health Care Policy Research guidelines)?
2. Analysis of nursing practice and education: Is the practice theory consistent with existing standards of education in nursing? Is the theory produced related to nursing diagnoses and nursing intervention practices?
3. Analysis of research: Is the practice theory supported by existing research internal and external to nursing?

The interrelationships of statements or propositions found in practice theory should also be addressed, perhaps using theoretical substruction (Dulock & Holzemer, 1991). Gaps and inconsistencies in the theory would thus become understood and problems with the adequacy of the theory become evident.

The internal analysis of practice theory can be approached by diagramming the sign (i.e., positive, negative, or unknown) of the interrelationship of all concepts found in the theory as described early by Hardy (1974). In this way, lapses and inconsistencies in the completeness of the concept structure can be addressed. Propositional adequacy of the overall theory is important, and at the practice level, it can be argued that more explicit statements, such as those that are necessary, sufficient, and directional in nature, are most important. Associational statements are also needed, but if they predominate, practice directions might not be adequately specific.

The internal analysis and evaluation of practice theory considers gaps and inconsistencies in the theory. In part, this is addressed by diagramming concepts and analyzing the propositions identified earlier. In addition, the overall theory is considered for problems involving completeness of thought and inconsistency of conclusions.

The assumptions of a given nation's theory of the historical and current perspectives of nursing are also considered. The current interpretations can be deduced from nursing models, which are of prime importance in determining whether nursing's historical perspective is evident. If there are conflicts with the practice theory and nursing's historical perspective, an assessment of the outcomes of the theory is needed. As with middle-range theory, practice theory could fit in nursing models that are themselves incongruent with each other; if this occurs, the choices made should be evident. Assumptions of practice theory are also relevant to a theory's ethical and cultural implications. Application of practice theory that conflicts with given cultural standards is arguably unethical. This assessment thus has practice application implications for nursing.

The external analysis and the evaluation of all levels of theory are currently "hot topics" because it is supported in EBP discussions and those of experiential knowledge must be assessed. Comparison of theory with the standards of practice, both external and internal to nursing, is an effort in this direction and is important to practice theory. Research in nursing and other areas is also examined, and the question of its support for the theory, its neutrality, or its opposition to the theory is evaluated.

In summary, the body of nursing knowledge within nations and between and among them is so extensive today that analysis and evaluation of all levels of theory are important—indeed necessary—for a valid and reliable approach to nursing care, research, and education. This is especially the case in cross-national nursing discussions; an interconnected body of knowledge in nursing in general cross-nationally might be possible for the first time in history; therefore, the discussion of an assessment of the fit between the levels of theory found in nursing cross-nationally needs to be addressed now.

With such assessment, nursing knowledge can be greatly expanded and clarified. Such assessment will at least lead to better understanding of the strengths and weaknesses of the nursing knowledge base and the identification of the parts of theory that need to be better developed. Analysis of each theoretical level should also lead to more knowledgeable "consumers" of nursing theory.

Middle-Range Theory (MRT)

MRT is particularly useful in research: It is sufficiently concrete to facilitate operationalization and is broad or abstract enough to facilitate general application. Merton (1977) discussed MRT at length and defined it as a theory lying somewhere between the most abstract ideas (e.g., grand theory-level nursing models) and more circumscribed concrete ideas (e.g., care procedures). Intervention research in nursing often produces MRT.

Merton (1977) stated that MRT can fall within or be congruent to several more abstract grand theories that are themselves incongruent with each other; thus, practice theories that are themselves incongruent with each other can fit in a given MRT. For example, decubitus ulcer care and practice theory might be congruent with two MRTs of elder care, which individually exhibit conflicting propositions and assumptions. MRT can be produced, therefore, by many methods (Walker & Avant, 1995). For example, there are "armchair" theorizing—theorizing from practice situations or more general phenomena—and developing an MRT by deductively generating statements from several existing theories (Whall, 1986).

The analysis and evaluation of MRT in this discussion use guidelines (or truth criteria) similar to those for analysis and evaluation of the conceptual nursing models. Although inherent in this level of theory, the metaparadigm concepts (person, environment, health, and nursing) have been eliminated from this analysis. Questions of more immediate relevance, such as the fit of the MRT with the existing cross-national nursing perspectives and domains, are asked. The more global metaparadigm concepts found in the models are not always implicit in MRT, although they can be inferred. Likewise, middle-range concepts have more specific empirical referents (or can be understood through human sense data) than the more abstract models.

TABLE 2–2   Criteria for Cross-National Analysis and Evaluation of Middle-Range Theory in a Given Nation

Basic Considerations
1. What are the definitions and relative importance of major concepts?
2. What are the type and relative importance of major theoretical statements and/or propositions?

Internal Analysis and Evaluation
1. What are the assumptions underlying the theory? What is the relationship to positions regarding the philosophy of science?
2. Are concepts related or not related via statements? Is there any resulting loss of information?
3. Is there internal consistency and congruency of all component parts of the theory?
4. What is the empirical adequacy of theory? Has it been examined in practice and research, and has it held up to this scrutiny?

External Analysis and Evaluation
1. What is the congruence between related theory and research internal and external to nursing?
2. What is the congruence with the perspective of nursing, the domains, and the persistent questions?
3. What ethical, cultural, and social policy issues are related to the theory?

Theoretical statements found in MRT can be categorized in part using Hardy's (1974) system or identified as ranging from causal to associative in nature. Theoretical statements or propositions of MRT should be assessed for their relative importance as well as for missing linkages between them. Theoretical substruction (Dulock & Holzemer, 1991), or the diagramming of all relationships found in a theory, can be used for this purpose. Missing relationships between concepts are also identified. For this purpose, a matrix is made of the sign of all the concepts; that is, one asks whether the relationship is positive, negative, or unknown. A decision is made about the relative importance of any missing concepts (i.e., whether missing data make the theory unclear).

Assumptions derived from the MRT are also analyzed by asking what is assumed to exist as the basis for the theory and what situation exists during the theory and after the theoretical action is concluded. Philosophy of science views is also discerned. Questions are asked about what the theory asserts to be true, what beliefs underlie the theory, and which positions in the philosophy of science the theory represents. These questions lead to further insights regarding congruence between statements and concepts of the theory.

The internal consistency (e.g., consistent use of terms) of MRTs is usually less a problem than that of more global discussions found in grand theories. Nevertheless, assessing all concepts to determine whether inconsistency in definitions occurs across the theory will assist in evaluating clarity. Empirical adequacy, the inherent ability to operationalize and measure aspects of a theory, is also important in MRT. Operational definitions are needed for empirical adequacy, and these too are evaluated (i.e., are they adequate and readily applied?).

External analysis of MRT involves congruence between global and MRT theories that are supported by research evidence and standards of practice. Even though MRT cannot directly guide practice, its relationship to professional practice is an important issue to consider.

Again, questions are also asked about each nation's nursing perspective: Is it represented consistently with the *historical* view (i.e., found in a nation's conceptual nursing models)? Because MRT is more readily applied than grand theory, its ethical, cultural, and social policies are crucial. Does the theory seem relevant to various cultural groups? Are there ethical concerns in this regard? What would be the result should social policy be based on this theory? Finally, assessment of the congruence of the perspective espoused by nursing with the domains of nursing that are currently accepted is determined: Where does the theory lead nursing? What research or other empirical examination is needed to more fully develop the theory?

NURSING CONCEPTUAL MODELS: ANALYSIS AND EVALUATION

The models of nursing and/or its grand theories examined here are likely to continue to have a major influence on nursing across nations. For example, products of the discipline such as nursing practice and research should be examined in light of nursing models that have been developed over a long period of nursing history in a given country. The conceptual nursing models are assessed from a postmodern view: That is, with the belief that these models are in and of themselves important, they are free to vary one from another, and they can be utilized as sources of either practice or MRT. Unlike those in disciplines in which grand theories do not continue to be influential, conceptual nursing models continue to guide various programs of research. The guidelines presented for these models highlight the differences and similarities of each model.

Historically, Dubin (1978) described grand theory–conceptual models as being composed of summative units, or abstract concepts; partial relationship statements or propositions usually join these concepts. Often the assumptions of the models are in essence the general beliefs or understanding of nursing theorists. The guidelines presented in Table 2–3, therefore, are not only for analysis but also for evaluation that students can continue to use as the model as it continues to be developed.

Because conceptual nursing models are composed of the major paradigm concepts found in the discipline (i.e., person, environment, health, and nursing) and concepts specific to the model, the first question to be

TABLE 2–3 Criteria for Cross-National Analysis and Evaluation of a Given Country's Nursing Conceptual Models

Introduction to the Model

Basic Paradigm Concepts Included in the Model

1. What are the definitions of *person, nursing, health*, and *environment?*
2. If there are additional understandings of *person*, what are they?
3. If there are additional understandings of *nursing*, what are they?
4. If there are additional understandings of *health*, what are they?
5. If there are additional understandings of *environment*, what are they?
6. What are the interrelationships among the concepts of person, nursing, health, and environment?
7. What are the descriptions of other concepts found in the model?

Internal Analysis and Evaluation

1. What are the model's underlying assumptions?
2. What are the definitions of any components of the model?
3. What is the relative importance of the model's basic concepts or other components?
4. What are the results of the analyses of internal and external consistency?
5. What are the analyses of adequacy?

External Analysis

1. Is nursing research based on the model or related to it?
2. Is nursing education based on the model or related to it?
3. Is nursing practice based on the model or related to it?
4. What is the relationship, if any, between existing nursing diagnoses and interventions systems?

asked often relates to the definition of these concepts. In addition to asking about the definition of *person* as defined throughout the model, the interrelationships of a person with the other concepts in the model are addressed. Often the way in which a person is discussed in different concepts related to the model fills out the description that the theorist wishes to give.

It is important to realize that although the term *person* is used in most of the models, the term *recipient of care* also could be used. This means that the recipient of care can be more than a single individual, for example, a family, a community, or a group with which a nurse is working.

It is important to understand whether *nursing* is used as a verb or as a noun according to the context in which it is used. The description of nursing in terms of the actions taken, of the goals of nursing, and of the view of society is addressed next. How this view is similar to or different from other commonly accepted views of nursing, such as those found in current organizations, is identified. Finally, the ways in which nursing addresses the care of individuals, families, groups, and communities are compared.

Health is addressed in each conceptual nursing model in overt or covert ways. Are the definitions and discussion of *health* given, is it seen as the goal of nursing, is its definition from another source used, and if there are various definitions of health, are they congruent with one another? If health is seen as some sort of steady state, are the propositional statements regarding health consistent with the steady-state perspective, or is health seen as an open, ever-evolving state that is related to all aspects of humans and their environment? The way in which the nurse acts to bring about health is of major interest to these analyses.

The way in which *environment* is defined is extremely important to nursing. Florence Nightingale, in essence, saw nursing as a science of environmental management. Her early emphasis on the environment brought to nursing the realization that there are physical and emotional environments as well as other types. It is of interest in the analysis to determine the way in which the theorist defines environment: Is it directional, linear, open, or closed; and is it interrelated with the other metaparadigm concepts?

The interrelationships among the four metaparadigm concepts are of interest because they identify the relative importance of each. For example, spending more time discussing person versus nursing in the model could result in some difficulty for practical applications of the model. If the interrelationships are of equal importance, is there some implied hierarchy as these concepts are addressed? The importance of these four major concepts can be fairly well determined by reading through all portions of the model to determine how each concept is described.

Additional concepts that describe the other elements of importance can be found in each model. Often, the other major concepts that the theorist uses actually define the model. The interrelationships among the major concepts of the model other than the four metaparadigm concepts must be addressed. Are they well defined? Are these relationships and their various outcomes described in detail? Is more detail needed?

The underlying assumptions on which the model is based are important in internal analysis and evaluation. They provide data about the nature of science ascribed to, for example, pragmatism or realism. The model's philosophical underpinnings should guide the relationship statements. In addition, whether there is conflict between the philosophical position suggested and the overall perspective of nursing should be determined. A part of the model analysis should address this.

Many times theories or subtheories are presented in a given nursing model. In what way are these or related elements congruent with the overall nursing model? For example, is a certain subtheory only identified but not further explored? If so, the model's internal and external consistency is affected because one would assume that this subtheory is of less importance.

Internal consistency has to do with the uniformity of discussion throughout the model. Are the concepts used in the same way when the model is initially determined as they are at the end? Are the propositional statements consistent with the model's assumptions? Are the propositional statements and concepts consistent with one another and with the assumptions of the model? Each of these points leads to a decision regarding the level of internal consistency.

External consistency must be addressed. For example, do the authors or theoreticians view the world in a manner consistent with views external to the model? Even though nursing models are not at a level that primarily suggests practice procedures, these questions are important. Likewise, is the model's view consistent with other conceptual nursing models, with other statements found in nursing, with elements such as the role of the nurse, and with nursing intervention classification systems? Each of these questions addresses the external consistency of the model.

Pragmatic adequacy is addressed; for example, does the model suggest feasible activities for nursing? Empirical adequacy asks, in essence, "Can model elements be measured?" The level of the model's abstraction certainly affects its usefulness and measurement: The more abstract the model, the more difficult it is to use and measure. If the concepts are highly abstract, it is often difficult to "bring them down" to a practice or more concrete level without using a good deal of interpretation. A nursing model with concepts that are much "rooted in the senses" or observable can, however, be difficult to relate back to its philosophical assumptions. Finally, the external analysis of the nursing model involves the way in which it has been used in research, education, and practice.

Although nursing diagnoses are not often stated in the nursing models, sections in every nursing model involve practice. Often these model sections lend themselves to nursing diagnoses that can be derived. These nursing diagnoses, however, cannot be congruent with external nursing diagnosis systems. For example, using Martha Rogers' model, one might identify a problem that is in an individual's environment. Although Rogers herself never used the term *nursing diagnosis* with her model, a diagnosis relating to the environment might be derived.

Not included here but a step related to derived nursing diagnoses is the identification of nursing interventions that are compatible with the nursing model (such as those found in NIC systems). Because the models presented here vary with respect to derivation of nursing diagnoses and interventions, it is left to the reader in many instances to determine possible diagnoses and interventions related to the model.

One important final note is that in this neomodernist era, some of the analytical and evaluative questions presented here might be less suitable for any one nation or even any one conceptual nursing model. When this occurs, the evaluative and analytic procedures outlined and discussed in this text can be useful for identifying various ways and means to produce or change whatever is needed in a given discipline of nursing. In this 21st century with its ever-increasing ready access between and among nations, cross-national differences in a discipline can seem daunting. These differences, however, also offer great hope as nations share their beliefs and ideas regarding nursing excellence.

REFERENCES

Abbey, R. (2000). Charles Taylor: Philosophy now. In J. Shand (Series Ed.), *Philosophy now*. Princeton, NJ: Princeton and Oxford Press.

Algase, D., & Whall, A. (1993). Rosemary Ellis' views on the substantive structure of nursing. *Image: Journal of Nursing Scholarship, 25*(1), 69–72.

Algase, D., & Whall, A. (1995, June). Analytic questions for emerging doctoral programs in nursing: An approach to develop culturally sensitive nursing content. *Proceedings, Nursing Forum on Doctoral Education*. Dearborn, MI: University of Michigan, School of Nursing.

Almutairi, A., & Rondney, P. (2013). Cultural competence for culturally diverse workforces: Toward equitable and peaceful health care. *Advances in Nursing Science, 36*(3), 200–212.

Arslanian-Engoren, C., Hicks, F., Whall, A., & Algase. D. (2005). An ontological view of advanced nursing practice. *Research and Theory for Nursing Practice, 10*(4), 315–322.

Baird, M. (2012). Well-being in refugee women experiencing cultural transition. *Advances in Nursing Science, 35*(3), 249–263.

Benner, P., Hooper-Kytiakidis, P., & Stannard, D. (1999). *Clinical wisdom and interventions in critical care: A thinking-in-action approach*. Philadelphia: W. B. Saunders.

Carper, B. (1978). Fundamental patterns of knowing in nursing. *Advances in Nursing Science, 1*(1), 13–23.

Donaldson, S. K., & Crowley, D. M. (1977). Discipline of nursing: Structure and relationship to practice. *Communicating Nursing Research, 10*, 1–22.

Dubin, R. (1978). *Theory building*. New York: Collier Macmillan.

Dulock, H., & Holzemer, W. (1991). Substruction: Improving the linkage from theory to method. *Nursing Science Quarterly, 4*(2), 83–87.

Hardy, M. (1974). Theories: Components, development, evaluation. *Nursing Research, 23*, 100–107.

Hunter, A., Wilson, L., Stanhope, M., Hatcher, B., Hattar, M., Messias, D., et al. (2013). Global health diplomacy: An integrative review of the literature and implications for nursing. *Nursing Outlook, 61*(2), 85–92.

Johnson, J., & Ratner, P. (1997). The nature of knowledge used in nursing practice. In S. Thorne & V. Hayes (Eds.), *Nursing praxis: Knowledge and action* (pp. 3–20). Thousand Oaks, CA: Sage.

Kim, H. S. (2011). *Foreword*. In P. G. Reed & N. B. Crawford, *Nursing knowledge and theory innovation: Advancing the science of practice*. New York: Springer, xi.

Lakatos, I. (1977). The methodology of scientific research programmes. In J. W. G. Currie (Ed.), *Philosophical papers* (Vol. 1). Cambridge: Cambridge University Press.

Laudan, L. (1977). *Progress and its problems*. Los Angeles: University of California Press.

McCarthy, G., & Fitzpatrick, J. J. (2012). *Leadership in action: Influential Irish women nurses' contribution to society*. Cork, Ireland: Oak Tree Press.

Merton, R. (1977). *On sociological theory*. New York: Free Press.

Phillips, D. C. (1987). *Philosophy, science, and social inquiry: Contemporary methodological controversies in social science and related applied fields of research.* New York: Pergamon Press.

Phoenix, P. (1964). *Realms of meaning.* New York: McGraw-Hill.

Reed, P. G. (1995). A treatise on nursing knowledge development for the 21st century: Beyond postmodernism. *Advances in Nursing Science, 17*(3), 70–84.

Reed, P. G. (1997). Nursing: The ontology of the discipline. *Nursing Science Quarterly, 10*(2), 76–79.

Schrag, C. O. (1997). *The self after postmodernity.* New Haven: Yale University Press.

Tasci-Duran, E., & Sevil, U. (2013). A comparison of the prenatal health behaviors of women from four cultural groups in Turkey: An ethnonursing study. *Nursing Science Quarterly, 26,* 257–266. doi:10.11770894318413489180

Walker, L., & Avant, K. (1995). *Strategies for theory construction in nursing.* Norwalk, CT: Appleton & Lange.

Whall, A. (1986). *Family therapy theory for nursing: Four approaches.* Norwalk, CT: Appleton & Lange.

Whall, A. (1989). The influence of logical positivism on nursing practice. *IMAGE: Journal of Nursing Scholarship, 21*(4), 243–245.

Whall, A. (2005). "Lest we forget": An issue concerning the Doctorate in Nursing Practice (DNP). *Nursing Outlook, 53*(1), 1.

Whall, A., & Hicks, F. (2002). The unrecognized paradigm shift within nursing: Implications, problems, and possibilities. *Nursing Outlook, 50*(2), 72–76.

Whall, A., Sinclair, M., & Parahoo, K. (2006). A philosophic analysis of evidence-based nursing: Recurrent themes, metanarratives, and exemplar cases. *Nursing Outlook, 54*(1), 30–35. doi:10.1016/j.outlook.2004.11.004

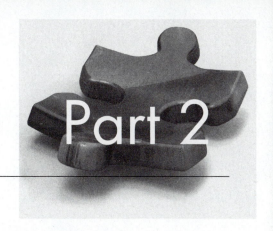

Part 2

Nursing Models from Other Countries

CHAPTER OUTLINE

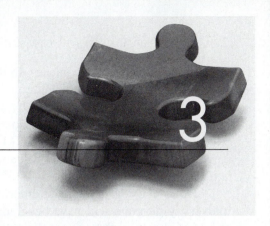

Australia: Shaping a Conceptual Model for the Registered Nurse: The Influence of the National Program Accreditation

Jill White

INTRODUCTION

This chapter focuses on the exploration of the extent to which the national accreditation council's standards for program accreditation shapes the conceptual framing of all national nursing curricula in Australia.

In July 2010, the new National Registration and Accreditation Scheme (NRAS) was introduced across Australia covering its six states and two territories (Department of Health, 2013). This necessitated the development of a single set of national standards for the accreditation of all nursing and midwifery programs leading to registration or higher endorsement with the new registration authority, the Nursing and Midwifery Board of Australia (NMBA). Prior to this legislative change, nursing registration and program accreditation had both been the province of state- and territory-based regulatory bodies, all of which were disbanded as part of the move to the new national registration body (NMBA) and a separate accreditation body, the Australian Nursing and Midwifery Accreditation Council (ANMAC) (Chiarella & White, 2013).

The necessity to produce new national guidelines provided an opportunity to develop ones that are pertinent to the contemporary Australian sociocultural and health contexts. In doing so, ANMAC mandated many areas of curriculum process and content that have direct implications for any conceptual model developed by a university to underpin its curriculum. The accreditation standards document "ANMAC Registered Nurse Accreditation Standards 2012" (ANMAC, 2012) details not only the nine specific standards but also significant contextual information within an extensive preamble (ANMAC, 1–7).

Every new registered nurse entering the profession from an Australian university program will have been educated following a curriculum that ANMAC has deemed to comply with its standards for accreditation. A direct consequence of this requirement to meet the standards is the premise that there are foundational elements common to all conceptual models in nursing education in Australia predetermined by these accreditation standards.

A brief explanation of the process of standards development is presented following a detailed exploration of the standards, revealing these predetermined conceptual elements.

THE PROCESS OF ACCREDITATION STANDARDS DEVELOPMENT

The development process of the standards for the registered nurse program accreditation was one of consensus building on a national level. An ANMAC working party of key stakeholders was convened to draft a first consultation document that was distributed to a wide range of relevant professional and government bodies and was placed on the Website with a public invitation for contribution. A large consultation forum was then held to distill the major issues and to form the basis of a second consultation paper. The second consultation paper and a draft of the new standards were then distributed. The working party considered all feedback and a final consultation forum was convened from which the penultimate version of the standards was determined.

The final version of the standards was then ratified by the ANMAC board and approved by NMBA as fulfilling the educational requirements for registration as required under the new NRAS law. The standards as published have the endorsement of all nursing and health professional bodies in Australia and the commonwealth, state, and territory ministers of health and can therefore be seen to represent consensus on the making of an "Australian registered nurse."

The role in this chapter's author in this process was to chair the working group, the Accreditation Advisory Committee, and the ANMAC board during the development and implementation of the standards. She was also the dean of a faculty that has used the new standards for program accreditation, and thus is a key informant on intention, process, and outcome in relation to the standards. Working group members are acknowledged at the end of this chapter.

Preamble to the Standards

With the predictable information in a preamble to a document such as this, which refers to the background, process, and purpose of the standards, there is a section that addresses two key areas, higher education reform and health systems reform. The changes in the tertiary education sector in Australia emphasize the educational quality assurance aspects of a program at a degree level or higher. More importantly with respect to conceptual framing are the references to the heath policy and health funding reforms in Australia. In part, the section on health reforms (ANMAC, 2012, 4) states:

> While the full impact of reforms is as yet unknown, the policy intent, at least at the Australian Government level is clear. There is a mandate for health services and health professionals to be more involved in **physical and mental health promotion and early intervention** to prevent progression of illness. Greater emphasis on providing services in **primary and sub-acute care settings** will be required along with the need for **stronger interprofessional awareness, collaboration and communication** to better support people with **complex illness and those who can self-care**. Facilitating transition from one health care setting to another is critical to reform success. So too is familiarity **with health informatics**, including person-controlled electronic health care records. The Australian Government's role as funder and program provider of aged care services flags emphasis on **accessible, seamless and comprehensive support for healthy ageing and care for older Australians** (emphasis added).

And this section of the preamble (ANMAC, 2012, 5) concludes by saying:

> it is likely that programs of study leading to registration as a registered nurse will require greater emphasis on **understanding the cost drivers** of health care as well as **enhanced knowledge of quality improvement, performance measurement and care coordination**. Broader experience and knowledge of **complex care, community, primary and sub-acute health care settings** are assumed under the National Health Reform Agreement. The education of nurses and other health professionals will require increased attention to developing the **knowledge, skills and emphasis to care for the elderly across the spectrum of wellness to ill health, particularly for those with dementia and multiple disease aetiologies**. Superior **communication and**

teamwork, delegation and supervision capabilities will be essential pre-requisites in the emerging health care environment. Also important will be the capacity to **innovatively use information technology and electronic resources to research the growing evidence base for improved care and treatment methods** (emphasis added).

The Standards

Nine standards for accreditation were developed. They include a standard on each of the following:

1. Governance
2. Curriculum conceptual framework
3. Program development and structure
4. Program content
5. Student assessment
6. Students
7. Resources
8. Management of workplace experience
9. Quality improvement and risk management

Criteria against which each standard is assessed were also developed and published (ANMAC, 2012).

Clearly, not all standards are equally pertinent to determining a conceptual model. Many are influential, but Standards 2, 3, and 4 (conceptual framework; program development and structure; program content, respectively) are of direct importance and in some areas, such as cultural competence, are quite prescriptive.

The four higher order concepts of the metaparadigm of nursing— nursing, person(s), health, and environment—will be addressed in order to capture the Australian ethos of nursing as predetermined by the accreditation authority. Whall's (2005) analysis and evaluation model will be used as the structuring device for this exploration; however, concepts will be explored in reverse order to usual order. The concepts developed through the explication of environment, health, and person(s) all compound to determine what the accreditation body expects as an Australian educated registered nurse and speak to the metaparadigm concept *nursing,* hence the reason for the reverse ordering.

ENVIRONMENT

The concept of *environment,* according to accreditation requirements, explicitly incorporates the essential geography and demography of Australia. There are direct references to the indigenous peoples and their health disparities, the multicultural nature of the population, the ageing of the nonindigenous population with simultaneous growth in the birth rate among Aboriginal and Torres Strait Islanders, and the disparity in health services between rural and remote areas and metropolitan areas.

Australia has a population of 23.5 million of whom 3% are Aboriginal or Torres Strait Islanders (Australian Bureau of Statistics, 2014). The country's indigenous history and culture are thought to be 50,000 years old; however, since colonization in 1788, there has been British/European dominance in law and government with its associated sociopolitical strengths and consequences. Aboriginal and Torres Straits Islander peoples have been permitted to vote only since 1962 and have been counted in national census data only since 1967. As a consequence of more than 100 years of unenlightened public policy, there are major disparities in health outcomes and educational opportunity between indigenous and nonindigenous populations (Burbank, 2011; McKenna, 2002). Australia enjoys the sixth highest life expectancy globally (Australian Institute for Health and Welfare, 2014a). Life expectancy at birth for a male infant born in 2012 is 79.9 years and for a female is 84.3 years; the life expectancy for Aboriginal and Torres Strait Islander babies born the same year is 10.6 years lower than the nonindigenous population for boys and 9.5 years lower for girls (Australian Institute for Health and Welfare, 2014a). Redressing this disparity is now a national priority with a raft of policy initiatives known as "closing the gap" initiatives (Council of Australian Governments, 2014).

Australia is a highly multicultural country with rapidly expanding legal immigration and a highly contested refugee policy for unanticipated arrivals. As of June 2013, 27.7% of residents were born overseas compared to 23.6% in 2003 and 10% in 1953, and 45% of Australians were either born overseas or have at least one parent born overseas (Australian Bureau of Statistics, 2014). The countries accounting for the highest influx, not surprising because of the country's history and geography, are the United Kingdom and New Zealand followed by China, India, Vietnam, the Philippines, and Italy (Australian Bureau of Statistics). Residents come from more than 200 countries, and more than 300 languages are spoken in Australian homes (Australian Bureau of Statistics).

As a consequence of, and in response to these demographics, the accreditation council mandates in the following standards (ANMAC, 2012, 14):

4.5 Inclusion of subject matter that gives students an appreciation of the diversity of Australian culture, develops their knowledge of cultural respect and safety, and engenders the appropriate skills and attitudes.

4.6 Inclusion of a discrete subject specifically addressing Aboriginal and Torres Strait Islander peoples' history, health, wellness and culture. Health conditions prevalent among Aboriginal and Torres Strait Islander peoples are also appropriately embedded into other subjects within the curriculum.

Cultural safety and cultural competence are therefore core elements of any concept of "nurse" in the Australian environment. Recognized as one of the key professional nursing bodies, the Congress of Aboriginal and Torres Strait Islander Nurses and Midwives has input into program development, provides guidelines on program content and process, and assists with access to cultural competence training for staff and students (Congress of Aboriginal and Torres Straits Nurses and Midwives, 2014). In the area of cultural competence, New Zealand has led and Australia has been a close follower (Wepa, 2005; Taylor & Guerin, 2010); cultural competence is now recognized as a fundamental nursing capability in many other countries. Fitzpatrick recognized the need for cultural competence in the United States in her editorial in 2007, and the publication of this book, which is a quest for culturally inclusive conceptual models, is further evidence of its growing importance (Fitzpatrick, 2007).

Geographically, the Australian population is both concentrated and dispersed. Of the population, 89% live in urban areas concentrated on the eastern coastal fringe; however, across the country, there are fewer than three persons per square kilometer (Australian Bureau of Statistics, 2014). The geographic spread of the population and the consequences for health and health service provision of distance and small and isolated population groups are of key importance to nurses. They not only make up the largest proportion of health care workforce but also are the mainstay of health service provision in rural and remote areas because of the extreme maldistibution of doctors in this country (Health Workforce Australia, 2012).

With the increase in Internet access and broadband width, the use of Telehealth and mobile technology has become an integral part of health care delivery, as have "paperless hospitals" and computers at the bedside. Nurses are now required to be educated to have sophisticated information technology capability in addition to their other well-developed professional skills.

The Australian society prides itself on its egalitarian nature. This is reflected in a legal system that values diversity and protects from discrimination. This protection has far-reaching implications for the education and practice of the nurse in relation to behavioral expectations and legal and ethical responsibilities.

HEALTH

The concept of *health* as shaped by accreditation is both broad and deep. Standard 2 specifies that curriculum processes and content incorporates "existing and emerging national and regional health priorities" (ANMAC, 2012, 14). National health priorities were first introduced federally in 1996 and are regularly reviewed. The introduction of new priorities is always an interesting signal of an area that can no longer be ignored. Australia has nine named national health priorities. Cancer, cardiovascular disease, injury prevention, and mental health were all introduced in the original 1996 grouping and have remained. The following were added sequentially: diabetes in 1997, asthma in 1999, arthritis and musculoskeletal conditions in 2002, obesity in 2008, and dementia in 2012 (AIHW, 2014b).

The list indicates a country with diseases of a developed, affluent society with an ageing and largely overweight population (63% is overweight or obese; AIHW, 2014b). The implications for nursing from this national priority list are obvious because these are diseases that require health promotion and illness prevention strategies and community-based chronic disease management because much, if not more than, of them focus on tertiary hospital care. Above all, people in need of services require an integration of health and social services that allows for the best care in the best environment.

In response to the health and illness demographics, the preamble to the standards explicitly mentions the emphasis needed for "primary health care and subacute care," "physical and mental health promotion," and "accessible, seamless and comprehensive support for healthy ageing and care for older Australians" (ANMAC, 2012, 4). An Australian notion of health is thus quite akin to the World Health Organization's definition of it as being a "state of complete physical, mental and social well-being and not merely the absence of disease or infirmity" (World Health Organization, 1948).

PERSON(S)

ANMAC accreditation standards say little directly about patients or people as the recipients of care. They speak, however, of the need for "highest patient care standards" (ANMAC, 2012, 20); the need "to improve patient access to health services, performance, transparency and accountability"; and "to better support people with complex illness and those who can self-care" (ANMAC, 4).

The standards document addresses the need for high levels of English language proficiency with English as the single official language of health care practice, which with the country's cultural and linguistic diversity, is necessary as a safety and quality issue for secure and effective communication.

"Professional collaboration" is frequently mentioned in the standards document and is inclusive of the person who is the recipient of care as an active participant in his or her care. This is reflected, albeit indirectly, through reference to "person-controlled medical records" (ANMAC, 2012, 4), "partnerships with Aboriginal and Torres Strait Islander health professionals and communities" (ANMAC, 11), and the idea of "collaboration and communication to better support people with complex illness and those who can self-care" (ANMAC, 4).

Despite the scarcity of direct comment on patients or person(s), there are many unspoken but well-understood indicators of the concept of *patient* or *person* that flow from the country's legal and ethical standards. Given the country's human rights legislation, the concept of *family* is defined as whatever the person considers it to be, no matter how conventional or unconventional. Competency assessment of a nurse's respectful, culturally proficient professional behavior is fundamental to the assessment of any educational program.

NURSING

The standards provide some explicit indications of expectations for the Australian educated registered nurse. Standard 2.1 specifies the requirement of a "clearly documented and explained conceptual framework for the program including educational and **professional nursing philosophies** underpinning its curriculum" (emphasis added) (ANMAC, 2012, 12). Standard 2.3 specifies the use of "contemporary and evidence-based approaches to professional nursing practice." Standard 2.4 refers to "integration of theory and practice, critical thinking and problem solving" skill development, "professional responsibility for continuing competence and life-long learning," and "use and learn from emerging research throughout their careers" and emphasizes developing "emotional intelligence," skills in "communication," "intra-professional and inter-professional learning for collaborative practice," "cultural safety," "ethical practice," and "leadership" (ANMAC, 12).

Standard 4.2 (ANMAC, 2012, 14) provides even more explicit direction:

> The central focus of the program is nursing practice, comprising core health professional knowledge and skills and specific nursing practice knowledge and skills that are evidence based, applied across the human

lifespan, and incorporate national and regional health priorities, health research, health policy and reform.

The preamble also emphasizes the nursing role in leadership and management of care and service provision: "a registered nurse will require greater emphasis on understanding the cost drivers of health care as well as enhanced knowledge of quality improvement, performance measurement and care coordination" (ANMAC, 2012, 4). "Superior communication and teamwork, delegation and supervision capabilities" are also professional expectations (ANMAC, 5).

These standards make clear that the Australian concept of nurse is one who is intellectually and professionally well developed, research focused, and committed to continuing competence with skills of inter- and intraprofessional collaboration and who is educated at a minimum at a degree level within the higher education sector.

A nurse is a leader in and manager and supervisor of the work of others in the care of people and the provision of health care; she or he must be culturally safe, a superior communicator, a skilled clinician, and technologically savvy and have a concept of nursing and care that is broader than the nurse–patient dyad. Nursing encompasses a sociopolitical understanding of health, illness, health services, and policy (White, 2014).

These standards and traits may seem highly aspirational, but with the complex demands of the country's health care environment and its geographic and demographic nature, Australia cannot afford to expect less of professional registered nurses. These traits therefore become part of the contextual concept of nurse and nursing in Australia and are mandated through processes of accreditation and assessed prior to registration.

The connection between and among concepts is, as noted, inferential. Expectations in relation to environment, health, and patient/person all inform the concept *nursing* and *nurse.* The explicit connection between and among concepts of the metaparadigm is made at the level of the individual curriculum and allows for institutional and regional differentiation within ANMAC's core expectations.

RELATIONSHIP TO NURSING AND HEALTH RESEARCH

The standards make several references to research as an underpinning to professional practice. They refer to evidence and research-based practice and research-led teaching. Research methodology and methods in nursing in Australia are of necessity broad and inclusive given the scope of knowledge that underpins any curriculum that would meet the standards. Ethical, personal, empirical, aesthetic, and sociopolitical knowing are all within the metaparadigm as shaped by the standards and require different forms of evidence and research (Fawcett, Watson, Neuman, Hinton, & Fitzpatrick, 2001; White, 1995).

RELATIONSHIP TO PROFESSIONAL PRACTICE

The national program standards are designed to ensure that each graduate of an accredited program has nursing practice as her or his central focus and that care is competently and seamlessly provided in multiple settings across health promotion; illness prevention; and subacute, acute, and critical care environments. The nurse is educated to have developed all national registered nurse competencies specified by the registration authority (NMBA, 2006) inclusive of a commitment to continuing competency, lifelong learning, and evidence-based, collaborative practice.

RELATIONSHIP TO NURSING EDUCATION

Not surprisingly, the standards present the greatest guidance in the area of education. As mentioned earlier, there are nine standards that address governance, resourcing, and quality processes (Standards 1, 7, and 9); the curriculum directly through conceptual framing, content, structure (Standards 2–4); and students, their workplace experience, and assessment of competency (Standards 5, 6, and 8).

The criteria for Standard 2 Curriculum Conceptual Framework (ANMAC, 2012, 12) provides these detailed educational expectations:

The program provider demonstrates:

2.1 A clearly documented and explained conceptual framework for the program, including the educational and professional nursing philosophies underpinning its curriculum.

2.2 The incorporation of contemporary Australian and international best practice teaching, learning and assessment methodologies and technologies to enhance the delivery of curriculum content, stimulate student engagement and promote understanding.

2.3 A program of study that is congruent with contemporary and evidence-based approaches to professional nursing practice and education.

2.4 Teaching and learning approaches that:
   a) enable achievement of stated learning outcomes
   b) facilitate the integration of theory and practice
   c) scaffold learning appropriately throughout the program
   d) encourage the application of critical thinking frameworks and problem-solving skills

   e) engender deep rather than surface learning
   f) encourage students to become self-directed learners
   g) embed recognition that graduates take professional responsi-
      bility for continuing competence and life-long learning
   h) instil students with the desire and capacity to continue to use,
      and learn from, emerging research throughout their careers
   i) promote emotional intelligence, communication, collaboration,
      cultural safety, ethical practice and leadership skills expected
      of registered nurses
   j) incorporate an understanding of, and engagement with, intra-
      professional and interprofessional learning for collaborative
      practice.

Such teaching and learning processes inevitably shape the concept formation of the learner/graduate.

SUMMARY AND CONCLUSION

This chapter originated from a serendipitous conversation between
Dr. J. Fitzpatrick and the author of this chapter when discussing this book
and the underlying assumption of country-specific or culturally relevant
conceptual models. Having lived and breathed the development of the new
accreditation standards in Australia, the author took this conversation as
a challenge to think about the extent to which the standards shaped or
predetermined core elements of any conceptual model in an Australian
curriculum. The exposition presented in this chapter is the outcome of an
invitation by Dr. Fitzpatrick to further that musing and to thoroughly inter-
rogate the standards to determine the extent to which ANMAC did indeed
delineate core aspects of an Australian nursing metaparadigm.

   The preceding analysis of each of the standards identifies the strong
influence of the Australian geography and demography, health priorities
and disparities, national legal and ethical frameworks, and social mores on
standards for registered nurse programs. Each of these standards in turn
focuses a national concept of nurse and nursing. This exposition demonstrates that intentionally or unintentionally, the accreditation council
through its standards for programs leading to registration as a nurse shapes
core notions of what it is to be a registered nurse in Australia and provides
the basis for a national conceptual model.

ANMAC RN Standards Working Party

      Ms. Amanda Adrian—CEO, ANMAC
      Ms. Julianne Bryce—Senior Federal Professional Officer, Australian
         Nursing Federation

Prof. Patrick Crookes—Chair, Council of Deans of Nursing and Midwifery

Ms. Leone English—ANMAC Board, Vocational Education and Training sector education provider

Ms. Joanna Holt—ANMAC Community Board member and project officer

Ms. Donna Mowbray—Director of Accreditation, Research, Innovation and Policy, ANMAC

Mr. Gordon Poulton—Director of Accreditation Services, ANMAC (July 2011 to January 2012)

Ms. Kathryn Terry—Accreditation Manager, ANMAC (July 2011 to April 2012)

Adjunct Prof. Debra Thoms—Member, Australian and New Zealand Council of Chief Nurses

Prof. Jill White—Chair, ANMAC Accreditation Advisory Committee, Chair ANMAC Board

REFERENCES

Australian Nursing and Midwifery Accreditation Council. (2012). *ANMAC registered nurse accreditation standards, 2012*. Canberra: Author. Retrieved from http://www.anmac.org.au/sites/default/files/documents/ANMAC_RN_Accreditation_Standards_2012.pdf

Australian Bureau of Statistics. (2014). *Australia's population*. Canberra: Author. Retrieved from http://www.abs.gov.au/AUSSTATS/abs@.nsf/Web+Pages/Population+Clock?opendocument#from-banner=LN

Australian Institute of Health and Welfare. (2014a). *Life expectancy*. Canberra: Author. Retrieved from http://www.aihw.gov.au/deaths/life-expectancy/

Australian Institute of Health and Welfare. (2014b). *National health priorities*. Canberra: Author. Retrieved from http://www.aihw.gov.au/national-health-priority-areas/

Burbank, V. (2011). *An ethnography of stress: The social determinants of health in aboriginal Australia*. New York: Plagrave McMillan.

Congress of Aboriginal and Torres Strait Island Nurses and Midwives. (2014). http://catsinam.org.au/

Chiarella, M., & White, J. (2013). Which tail wags which dog? Exploring the interface between health professional regulation and health professional education. *Nurse Education Today, 33,* 1274–1278. Retrieved from http://www.nurseeducationtoday.com/article/S0260-6917(13)00046-4/fulltext

Council of Australian Governments. (2014). *Closing the gap in indigenous disadvantage*. Canberra: Australian Government. Retrieved from https://www.coag.gov.au/closing_the_gap_in_indigenous_disadvantage

Department of Health. (2013). *National registration and accreditation scheme, 2010*. Canberra: Australian Government. Retrieved from http://www.health.gov.au/internet/main/publishing.nsf/Content/work-nras

Fawcett, J., Watson, J., Neuman, B., Hinton, P., & Fitzpatrick, J. (2001). On nursing theories and evidence. *Journal of Nursing Scholarship, 33*(2), 115–119.

Fitzpatrick, J. (2007) Cultural competence in nursing education revisited. *Nursing Education Perspectives, 28*(1), 5.

Health Workforce Australia. (2012). *Australia's future health workforce (HW2025).* Adelaide: Author. Retrieved from https://www.hwa.gov.au/our-work/health-workforce-planning/health-workforce-2025-doctors-nurses-and-midwives

McKenna, M. (2002) *Looking for blackfella's point: An Australian history of place.* Sydney: UNSW Press.

Nurses and Midwives Board of Australia. (2006). *Registered Nurse Competency Standards.* Melbourne: Author. Retrieved from http://www.nursingmidwiferyboard.gov.au/Codes-Guidelines-Statements/Codes-Guidelines.aspx#competencystandards

Taylor, K., & Guerin, D. (2010). *Health care and indigenous Australians: Cultural safety in practice.* South Yarra, Victoria. AUS: Palgrave McMillan.

Wepa, D. (2005). *Cultural safety in Aotearoa New Zealand.* Auckland, NZ: Pearson Education New Zealand.

Whall, A. (2005). The structure of nursing knowledge. In J. Fitzpatrick & A. Whall (eds.). *Conceptual models of nursing: Analysis and application* (4th ed.). Upper Saddle River, NJ: Prentice Hall.

White, J. (1995). Patterns of knowing: Review, critique and update. *Advances in Nursing Science, 17*(4), 73–86.

White, J. (2014). Through a socio-political lens: The relationship of practice, education, research, and policy to social justice. In P. Kagan, M. Smith & P. Chinn (eds.) *Philosophies and practices of emancipatory nursing: Social justice as praxis.* New York, NY: Routledge, 298–308.

World Health Organization. (1948). *WHO definition of health.* Geneva: Author. Retrieved from http://www.who.int/about/definition/en/print.html

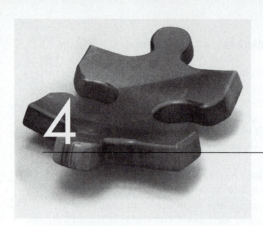

4

Canada: Strengths-Based Nursing: A Value-Driven Approach to Practice

Laurie N. Gottlieb and Norma Ponzoni

INTRODUCTION

Strengths-based nursing (SBN) blends both old and new approaches to nursing. It is "old" inasmuch as SBN reconnects with Florence Nightingale's vision. The new elements represent a shift away from the dominant deficit, problem-based health care model (Gottlieb, 2013).

In 1860, Nightingale published her seminal book on nursing, *Notes on Nursing*, in which she laid out her vision for modern secular nursing. She envisioned nursing's mandate as health and healing, and the nurse's role was "to put the patient in the best condition for nature to act on him" (Nightingale, 1860, 133). Nightingale believed that humans possessed innate growth as well as restorative and repair capacities (i.e., strengths) that nurses needed to understand and work with to promote health and facilitate healing.

Most nursing models follow the traditional medical model that concerns ascertaining problems and then fixing them. Concerns and issues are viewed through a *deficit and pathological lens*. There is a preoccupation with what is lacking, missing, or not functioning. However, deficits are only one aspect of a person's total being. SBN does *not* negate or ignore problems, but it does require the nurse to understand the whole person in the context of his or her environments, both physical and relational, as well as historical and the many aspects of his or her life. SBN focuses on what is functioning and what the person does best in order to maximize his or her health and healing. SBN is characterized by four key concepts.

Key Concept 1: SBN Is an Approach to Nursing Guided by Core Values

SBN is *not* a model but an approach to nursing built on a strengths-based philosophy that subscribes to a set of eight core values to guide action. SBN is a state of consciousness or way of thinking that guides the way in which the nurse responds to patients. SBN uses positive, holistic, person-centered, *empowering* language that is consistent with this approach, which includes working with a person's strengths to deal with problems, manage deficits, and minimize weaknesses. This chapter elaborates on each of these values as they pertain to health, person, environment, and nursing.

In addition, a *strengths-based nursing* approach is consistent with patient and family-centered care (Morgan & Yoder, 2012).

Strengths.   In SBN, strengths exist at all levels from cell (biological), to citizen (whole person), to community. *Strength* is an umbrella term that includes both the internal qualities of a person or unit (family, community) and the external resources available to the person or unit. Strengths include a person's and family's assets, attitudes, attributes, capacities, competencies, resources, skills, talents, and traits that define a person's uniqueness and enable him or her to function at maximum capacities (Gottlieb, 2013). Strengths are the things a person does best: what works, and functions. These concepts also apply at the family and community levels.

In caring for a person, the nurse uncovers and discovers strengths and then capitalizes on them or develops new ones, enabling the person to achieve higher levels of health or to heal.

Key Concept 2: SBN Capitalizes on Innate Capacities of Health and Innate Mechanisms of Healing

People are born with capacities that enable them to grow, develop, and flourish (i.e., become healthy, integrated individuals) as well as the mechanisms to repair and restore (i.e., self-heal). Examples of health capacities include inborn hardware to connect and develop attachments; to regulate physiologically processes, emotions, and cognitive or thought processes; to cope with stress; and to develop agency (autonomy). Examples of repair and restorative mechanisms include neurogenesis (neuronal repair and rerouting), immunological responses to foreign agents (pathogens and mutations), circadian rhythms such as sleep-wake cycles, and extensive pathways that connect the brain and the nervous and immune systems. These health capacities and healing mechanisms can be developed, modified, and affected by experience, quality of human interactions, and environments (Schweitzer, Gilpin, & Frampton, 2004). Moreover, new capacities, competencies, and skills can be acquired through learning. These health capacities and healing mechanisms are a person's greatest assets and constitute her or his inner and outer strengths. Because they appreciate that working with strengths is key to health (i.e., becoming) and healing, SB nurses look to uncover and discover a person and a family's inner and outer strengths. Nurses create conditions to strengthen and support existing strengths or to help a person/family acquire new strengths. When innate strengths are compromised, threatened, or not fully developed, nurses can compensate for (e.g., do for), supplement (e.g., provide nutrients), scaffold (e.g., help with), protect (e.g., reduce risk), and/or create healing environments (e.g., physical surroundings). These acts are performed within the context of a therapeutic nurse–patient relationship in which the nurse is authentically engaged (see Key Concept 4).

Key Concept 3: SBN Is Built on Principles of Empowerment

SBN recognizes the power of people who believe that they can exercise control over their lives and health care decisions (Rodwell, 1996). These people derive power from recognizing possibilities and creating opportunities, being able to make choices, and feeling empowered within themselves to effect change. People must empower themselves (Gibson, 1991). However, nurses can create conditions that enable someone to become self-empowered. Focusing on a person's strengths enables him or her to become motivated and provides her or him with the energy to make choices, take action, and be in charge (Miller & Rollnick, 2002). When nurses create these conditions, people respond with hope and a greater sense of well-being. This approach of empowerment is very different from the deficit model that relies on the negative and the fear, uncertainty, and denial (FUD) factors to secure compliance or deal with problems. Finally, SB nurses understand that they are not in the business of "fixing" problems.

Key Concept 4: SBN Is a Set of Relational/Moral/and Social Activities with a Technical Basis

SBN recognizes that humans are wired to connect with one another (Lieberman, 2013) but not to relate to machines. With increasing reliance on technology to diagnose and treat symptoms, disease, and disabilities, care has become fragmented and depersonalized and patients objectified. Nursing is far too often practiced as a set of technical activities and tasks than as a set of relational activities with a technical basis (Steele & Harmon, 1979).

SBN reaffirms that the core of nursing is the nurse–patient relationship and that the effectiveness of nursing rests in establishing a trusting, empathetic relationship. It is through connecting with patients and families that nurses can create conditions for growth, healing, and transformation (Newman, 2008).

SBN: DEFINITION AND DESCRIPTION OF THE CONCEPTS WITHIN NURSING'S METAPARADIGM

The definition and description of *health, person, environment, and nursing* are embodied in the values that make up the SBN approach. It should be noted that describing SBN in the context of nursing's metaparadigm is useful as a theoretical exercise to highlight the differences between the SBN approach and those nursing models that are deficit based.

SBN is considered a paradigm shift from the deficit, disease, and oriented models because it derives from a different set of assumptions, subscribes to a different way of thinking and a new set of values and principles, and uses strengths-based language. In practice, the four components of nursing's metaparadigm are indivisible and must be considered as a unitary whole.

At the core of SBN are the following assumptions as they relate to *health, person, environment, and nursing* (Gottlieb, 2013, 57):

- Individuals, families, and communities aspire to and are motivated to have better health and healing.
- Persons have the capacity to grow, transform, and self-heal.
- Inherent within all things from cells, to citizens, and to communities are potentials and strengths.
- Problems, weaknesses, vulnerabilities, hardships, and suffering are parts of the human condition.
- Strengths are required for health and self-healing.
- Within each person resides the power to self-heal, which is in itself a strength.
- Strengths enable people to adapt to different environments and cope with life experiences to meet a wide range of health challenges.
- Environments contain powerful forces that select for specific strengths or deficits that will determine how a person survives and grows or withers in a particular environment.

- Nursing exists to create conditions that enable a person's innate and acquired strengths to function at his or her maximum capacity to enable the person to achieve greater health and facilitate healing by alleviating his or her physical and emotional suffering.
- Nursing works with people and their environments to select for and develop strengths to promote health and facilitate healing.

Definition and Description of Health and Healing

Health and healing are among SBN's eight core values guiding nurses' actions. Health and healing are viewed as two distinct but interrelated concepts. Health is about creating wholeness; healing is about restoring wholeness (Gottlieb, 2013). These concepts are described separately and then discussed in relationship to one another.

Health.
A separate entity that coexists with disease, trauma, and injury (Allen, 1977; Cowling, 2000), *health* is a distinct entity irrespective of the extensiveness or severity of the disease, condition, or injury. One can have health even at the end of life.

Inspired by Nightingale's concept of health as "becoming" (Nightingale, 1860), SBN considers health to be the process by which one creates wholeness and becomes an integrated self (Gottlieb, 2013) in order to be able to adapt with flexibility to ever-changing environments and conditions (Siegel, 2012). Indicators of health can include capacities to lead meaningful, purposeful, and satisfying lives, create meaningful and secure relationships, effectively regulate physiological and emotional arousal levels, and rally in a timely manner from insults and learn from them to achieve higher levels of becoming (Gottlieb, 2013; Gottlieb & Gottlieb, 2007).

Humans are born with innate capacities that can be considered the building blocks or potential strengths in the process of becoming—from healthy fetus to healthy child to healthy adult. Wholeness is created through the development of these innate capacities and competencies and the acquisition of skills to deal with life's challenges, find purpose, and get the most out of living. These capacities, competencies and skills are both inherited and acquired. They are designed to be modified by experience, environments, and culture. These building blocks or innate capacities for health (i.e., potential strengths) include the capacity to form attachments (relating and connecting to others), regulate physical and emotional arousal levels, engage in executive planning, cope with stress (Gottlieb & Gottlieb, 2007), strive for competence to be agenic (Deci & Ryan, 1985), and have the capacity to learn. Through age, maturation, and experience, embodied and embedded aspects of the whole person become increasingly well organized, coordinated, and integrated (Siegel, 2012).

Healing. Most nursing models subsume *healing* under health because they conceptualize health on a continuum and define it as the absence of disease. Thus, at the far end of the continuum is poor health that therefore requires healing. According to SBN, health coexists with disease and is a separate entity, so healing must be considered as a distinct but interrelated entity with health.

Inspired by Nightingale's ideas on healing, it is viewed as a reparative and restorative process (Nightingale, 1860). Humans are wired for innate repair and growth mechanisms that result in healing. These mechanisms reside in a body's physiological system such as the neurological and immunological. In the process of healing (i.e., restoring wholeness), the embodied person "learns" and rallies from insults (Audy, 1971). Learning involves responding to acquired information, which occurs at many levels such as the cellular, organismal, family, and community. Through healing and recovery, people can attain new levels of health.

Definition and Description of Person

SBN's units of concern can be the individual, the family, the community, or any combination of these three, depending on the presenting issue and its context. For example, if the nurse and family identify that the issue is a family one, then the family becomes the unit of concern and the nurse considers how individual family members and/or friends or the community interface with, influence, and are being influenced by the family.

Of the eight core SBN values, five SBN values define and describe the *person:*

1. Uniqueness
2. Holism and embodiment
3. Subjective reality and created meaning
4. Self-determination
5. Learning, readiness, and timing

Uniqueness of the Person. This value refers to the distinctiveness of each individual, family, and community. No two entities are alike because no two people (even identical twins) share the same genetic/biological makeup, inheritance patterns, experiences, culture, and so on. Uniqueness exists at all levels: biologic, person, family, and so forth. Although humans share many universal capacities and experiences that can enable them to relate to another's suffering and respond with a common humanity, each person and every family are more different than similar when humans consider individuals (Harris, 2006). Each individual responds to and reacts in his or her own specific, idiosyncratic, unique way.

Uncovering and understanding what makes a person unique and defines her or his "specialness" provides nurses a window through which to view that person's strengths. The corollary is also the case. Often by understanding her or his strengths, a person's uniqueness is revealed. People's uniqueness is reflected in their responses to health and healing as well as to how they cope with life's challenges, both ordinary and extraordinary. This uniqueness is also reflected in how they respond to medical treatments and clinical interactions.

Holism and Embodiment of the Person. This SBN value speaks to the idea that a person is an integrated, unitary being who functions as an indivisible whole (Rogers, 1970). The *person* is both embodied inasmuch as the mind and body are one and embedded in relationships and in the context of their lives (Siegel, 2012). Both the body and mind are "knowers" and respond in a unitary way (Benner & Wrubel, 1989).

Subjective Reality and Created Meaning of the Person. The third value is intertwined with the value of uniqueness. Because human beings have a unique biological constitution and experience their environments in their own ways, each person attends to, attunes to, and then selects from aspects of his or her many meaningful environments. From these experiences, human beings create their own reality that in turn affects how they see, think, and behave. As part of making sense of and understanding their many life worlds, individuals and families must interpret events. One way to create meaning is by developing narratives. It is in these narratives that the nurse comes to understand how individuals perceive and experience their worlds.

Self-Determination of the Person. The fourth value speaks to the underlying idea of the agenic nature of humans. Humans strive for autonomy and for being agenic, that is, taking charge of their lives including making decisions that affect their health (Deci & Ryan, 1989). SBN believes that along with being agenic, people change when they are actively involved in making decisions and choices that best fit who they are and that are consistent with their beliefs and values and the nature of their circumstances in order to feel in control.

Learning, Readiness, and Timing of the Person. As to the fifth value, *learning* refers to the changes that affect behavior and can occur at many levels including neurobiological (Cozolino, 2013). The innate capacity to learn enables a person to acquire the competencies and skills to navigate through life's events both small and large; these competencies and skills are also needed for health and healing. Illness, adversity, and trauma challenge the person but at the same time can be opportunities for growth and transformation. The latter is possible through learning. It is in the course of dealing with adversity that inner and outer strengths are revealed and are developed.

Learning depends on readiness and timing. *Readiness* occurs when a person is primed to learn and change; *timing* refers to when a change is most likely to occur (Gottlieb, 2013). When timing and readiness are optimal, a person becomes an active learner, seeking the knowledge and skills needed to cope and adapt.

Definition and Description of Environment

Florence Nightingale (1860) sensitized nurses to the importance of the environment and its role in health and healing. Thus, understanding environments and working with them is a central idea of SBN. Environments can be modified and the role of nursing is to create those that "put the patient in the best condition" by promoting health and facilitating healing. Environments can be physical, interpersonal, cultural/social, and political.

Another core SBN value is that the *person and environment are integral.* Each shapes and is shaped by the other and is in constant and continuous transactions. In effect, person and environment are inseparable. The discussion of environments is complex and vast (Gottlieb, 2013). For the purpose of this chapter, a number of features of environments are highlighted.

First, environments can be internal and external. *Internal environments* refer to tissue microenvironments that include cells, tissues, extracellular lymphatic, cardiovascular fluids, and the like.

External environments are physical, interpersonal, cultural/social, and political.

- *Physical environments* include the quality and size of the healing space. Such elements as design, décor, layout, air quality, ventilation, setting, and people density are some of the features that affect health and healing (Schweitzer et al., 2004).
- *Interpersonal environments* comprise all interactions, transactions, connections, and relationships. The quality of a person's interpersonal relationships is a major determinant of health. Nurses play an integral part in a person's interpersonal environment. Every encounter, every interaction, and every nonverbal and verbal

gesture (both direct and indirect, near and at a distance) have the power to heal and to cause harm.

- *Culture* shapes a person's thoughts, feelings, values, and beliefs. A person's culture helps to understand his or her person.

Second, environments are experienced in subjective ways. Individuals attend to and select those aspects of the environment that are relevant and significant. The timing of events affects whether a person processes what is happening in his or her environment and how he or she interprets and makes meaning of the event.

Third, environments are nested in systems and different cultures that affect individuals and families to varying degrees, directly and indirectly (Bronfenbrenner, 1979). For example, families are nested in neighborhoods, in towns or cities, in states and national political cultures, in a society in a larger global network, and so forth. People are affected by the system they come into direct contact and interact with that in turn is affected by the systems in which those systems are nested. For example, when people are sick, a hospital's environment will affect their ability to heal. Just as the hospital environment exerts an influence, so too do health care policies and insurance health care coverage.

Fourth, people do best in environments where there is a "goodness-of-fit." This occurs when people have the capacities to meet the challenges of their environment and when the environment adapts to and brings out the best in those people. When this is the case, there is a positive transaction between a person and her or his environment as she or he is able to meet the demands and expectations put on each person. However, when an environment is too challenging or nonsupportive, a person can become overwhelmed, and the environment can be a poor fit and become toxic.

Definition and Description of Nursing

Nursing has a unique social mandate and obligation to society. Its social contract is to promote health by creating conditions for people to "become" and realize their fullest potential, to heal and recover from insults and injuries, and to alleviate suffering brought about by disease, accidents, and trauma. Because humans have capacities for health and innate mechanisms to heal themselves, nurses need to know and understand these capacities and mechanisms and how to assess and work with them.

In order to create conditions for health and healing, a nurse is guided by the eight SBN core values. The nurse uses these values to get to "know" a person and his or her personhood, circumstances, strengths, problems, issues, concerns, environments, and the like that influence him or her.

The nurse uses the *spiraling process* with its four phases (i.e., exploring, zeroing in, working on, and reviewing) to assess a patient, and, in the process, to discover the person's innate and acquired inner and outer strengths (Gottlieb, 2013, Chapter 9). The nurse then creates conditions to assist the person to self-heal by working to develop strengths or to turn deficits into strengths (Gottlieb, 2013, Chapter 10).

SBN considers the nurse to be the instrument for health and healing and the one who creates the conditions for healing through the quality of transactions with patients and families and by establishing a trusting, open, and nonjudgmental relationship. A nurse uses his or her caring attributes of compassion and authentic presence to create secure and supportive environments. By using knowledge from the biological, social, and nursing sciences, the nurse is able to help patients and families develop and acquire strengths that will enable them to find solutions to their problems (McAllister, 2003). An example is a situation in which the nurse helps to control the patient's pain. The nurse in effect is creating conditions to promote rest and sleep and to redirect energy toward the body's immunological system, thereby supporting the body's innate mechanisms to heal.

Nurses learn how to create conditions by retraining their senses in the art and science of nursing (Gottlieb, 2013, Chapter 6). Nursing involves developing skills of clinical inquiry and of skilled know-how in carrying out medical and nursing acts (Bennerr, Hooper-Kyriakidis, & Stannard, 2011) by becoming astute observers and learning to listen attentively (Gottlieb, 2013, Chapter 7 and 8).

Because the power to heal is innate and the power to manage one's own care resides in the person and family, the nature of the nurse–patient relationship is one in which both the nurse and person need to become fully engaged by developing a *collaboration partnership*. This is a nonhierarchical relationship in which the nurse shares power with the patient (Gottlieb & Feeley, 2006) and works "with" the person rather than just "does" for her or him. To share power, the nurse recognizes the importance of the person's being able to take charge of her or his life and make decisions. Whereas the nurse possesses knowledge and expertise in health and healing matters, she or he recognizes that the person and the family possess knowledge of himself or herself, his or her life history and circumstances and can develop skills that can be critical in his or her own self-healing. The nurse assumes the role of learner and looks to the person and family to teach her or him. When the nurse has relevant knowledge to impart or skills that the patient needs to learn to be able to care for himself or herself, the nurse is the teacher and the person is the learner. Patients are more likely to engage as partners when they come to believe in themselves and know that they have something to bring to the relationship. They often arrive at this awareness when the nurse identifies those areas of their personhood that are their strengths.

Nursing from a strengths-based approach requires a nurse to have specific qualities that must be developed, or if they exist, reinforced and deepened. Essential nurse qualities fall into four sets of strengths including (a) strengths of mind-set (e.g., mindfulness, nonjudgmental, humility), (b) strengths of knowledge and knowing (e.g., curiosity, self-reflection), (c) strengths of relationship (e.g., trustworthiness, empathy, compassion), and (4) strengths of advocacy (e.g., self-efficacy, courage) (see Gottlieb, 2013, Chapter 5).

ANALYSIS AND EVALUATION

Relationship Among Concepts and Components of the Strengths-Based Nursing Approach

SBN is based on a strengths-based philosophy that has as its bedrock principles of empowerment, health promotion, person-centered care, and collaborative partnership (Gottlieb, 2013). The eight core values that compose an SB approach are highly interrelated and integrated. Only when these values are used together do they form a holistic approach to guide nurses in creating conditions for health and healing.

The eight values guide the nurse to create conditions for people to become self-empowered by mobilizing, capitalizing, and developing the person and family's inner and outer strengths. To empower oneself requires that a person develop an attitude and a belief in himself or herself and have the power within and the outer resources that are capable of attaining and preserving health with abilities to restore, repair, renew, and, in some instances, even recover through innate mechanisms and processes of healing. These people also have the capacities to develop knowledge and acquire skills to take charge and to know where they can exercise control to achieve their goals and bring about the desired change. In so doing, they engender within themselves and others feelings of hope and a renewed sense of purpose and become motivated to achieve their goals.

Nurses put patients in the "best condition" by attending to the fundamentals of health and healing (e.g., exercise, hygiene, sleep, nutrition, stress management, pain management). Nurses accomplish this by supporting the body's healing mechanism by attending to the fundamentals of safety (e.g., physical safety, infection control, creation of a safe physical environment) and by working collaboratively with physicians and the health care team to carry out medical treatments, procedures, and the like. Nurses work to support and enlarge the inner and outer strengths (e.g., biological, psychological, social, financial) of the person, family, and community. This work can involve reinforcing and supporting existing strengths, working to develop a patient's potential, and turning deficits into strengths (Gottlieb, 2013). These nursing activities engage the patient within the context of a trusting relationship.

Relationship to SBN and Health Research

Evidence regarding SBN's effectiveness comes from many bodies of research, biological, social, and nursing sciences. An extensive body of research from positive psychology supports many of the concepts inherent in SBN, such as the role of empowerment, self-efficacy, and hope, and recognize its contributions to health, harmony, and well-being (Lopez & Snyder, 2011; Snyder & Lopez, 2009).

SBN is relational, and evidence of the efficacy of the importance of supportive, compassionate relationships to health and healing come from the newly emerging field of interpersonal neurobiology (Siegel, 2012), the vast research on social support (Thiots, 2011), the growing body of evidence from attachment theory (Cassidy & Shaver, 2008), and nursing science (Bluvol & Ford-Gilboe, 2004; see also the *Annual Review of Nursing Research* series published by Springer).

SBN is holistic and embodied. Evidence of the importance of the mind–body connection in promoting or interfering with innate mechanisms of healing derives from the fields of psychoneurobiology and stress and coping (Aldwin & Park, 2007; Lanius, Bluhm, & Frewen, 2011).

Finally, SBN has evolved from the McGill model of nursing (Gottlieb & Rowat, 1987) that has been shown to improve health when nurses focus on strengths and opportunities (e.g., Ford-Gilboe, 2000; Pless, Feeley, Gottlieb, Dougherty, & Willard, 1994). A meta-analysis of nurse-led interventions that provided comprehensive, patient-centered care found that this approach resulted in better health outcomes at cost savings compared with the approach when nurses' primary focus was medical or deficit based (Browne, Birch, & Thabane, 2012).

Relationship to Nursing Education

A strengths-based approach in education is known as *strengths-based teaching and learning* (SBTL) (Gottlieb & Gottlieb, 2013; Gottlieb & Benner, 2013) and is guided by the same values of practice.

SBN believes that nursing is a lifelong learning pursuit and that nurses need to be committed to updating their knowledge and developing new skills if they are to have the flexibility to adapt to new conditions and changing demands.

Nursing educators whose philosophy of practice is strengths based extend this philosophy to their pedagogy. Strengths-based thinking and being are just as relevant when the unit of concern is the learner. Just as nurses are concerned with creating conditions for a patient's health and healing, educators create learning environments to enable students to achieve their goals as professionals.

SBTL focuses on retraining the senses for learning to nurse at a basic and advanced level, developing the skills of clinical inquiry and of sound decision making, acquiring new knowledge, and developing competencies and technical skills to become expert practitioners, administrators, educators, and researchers.

Educators who adopt an SBTL approach serve as role models and through their actions demonstrate what SBN is. The teacher becomes a living exemplar of the possibilities that SBN affords. Students come to understand at a deeper level the empowering effect of SBN compared to a deficit, critical approach.

Relationship to Professional Practice

SBN operationalizes person-family centered care that deeply respects patients and families and gives both the dignity they require to heal. SBN blends science, patient experiences, and frontline nurses' experiences in caring for patients and families.

Nurses whose framework of practice has been strengths based have been essential in developing this approach to care. These nurses have shared insights and told stories of the benefits of working with person and family strengths and have made visible their work and the knowledge and skilled know-how that are involved in SBN (Gottlieb, 2013; Gottlieb & Feeley, 2006). Patients and families have also recounted how this nursing approach has made the difference (Ezer, Bray, & Gros, 1997).

SBN fits with practice because it uses language that is derived from nurses who practice from a strengths perspective. SBN captures what expert nurses have come to know as their best practice (Benner as cited in Gottlieb, 2013). By putting the elements together, SBN gives nurses a framework, an orientation, and a language to describe the nature of their work not only to themselves but also to their patients, other nurses, colleagues, employers, and the public.

In today's health care environment with the complexity of patient situations, patients and families benefit from the knowledge and expertise of all health care professionals. However, a multidisciplinary approach works only when each member of the team has a unique set of skills and knowledge and the training and education to use them. Even though the edges among professionals may be blurred, nonetheless each profession and each discipline must contribute something that is uniquely its own in order to be relevant and held accountable for their actions and practices (Gottlieb & Gottlieb, 1998). SBN gives nursing a distinct role in the health care system that complements but does not duplicate or replace medicine. With its focus on relational care, SBN's uniqueness lies in its holistic, integrative approach to practice with its focus on creating conditions to maximize the innate healing of a person and family by tailoring care in partnership with them that best fits them and their situation and circumstances.

For nurses to be able to practice SBN, they should seek education in institutions, agencies, and units that subscribe to SBN values. Nurse leaders and managers need to create healthy workplace environments that provide the support and tools to practice autonomously to the full scope of their knowledge and skills. This happens when an institution or agency adopts strengths-based care as its philosophy and when nursing leaders and managers are guided by SBN principles and values (Gottlieb, Gottlieb, & Shamian, 2012).

CONCLUSION

With the health care system in flux, there is a unique opportunity for nurses to reclaim nursing and by doing so, to improve the health of people. Nursing and nurses have not been given the power or accorded the recognition commensurate with their central role in the health care system. SBN, which has the power to change this imbalance, highlights nursing's distinct contribution to health and healing that complements medicine. In so doing, SBN gives nurses a voice, and with that voice, a stronger identity and pride in being nurses. They can play a key role in transforming health care.

ACKNOWLEDGEMENTS

Dr. Bruce Gottlieb for his invaluable assistance in preparing this chapter.

REFERENCES

Aldwin, C. M., & Park, C. L. (2007). *Handbook of health psychology and aging.* New York: Guilford Press.
Allen, M. (1977). Comparative theories of the expanded role in nursing and its implications for nursing practice: A working paper. *Nursing Papers, 9*(2), 38–45.

Audy, J. R. (1971). Measurement and diagnosis of health. In P. Shepard & D. McKinley (Eds.), *Environmental essays on the planet as a home* (pp. 140–157). Boston: Houghton Mifflin.

Benner, P., & Wrubel, J. (1989). *The primacy of caring: Stress and coping in health and illness.* Menlo Park, CA: Addison-Wesley.

Benner, P., Hooper-Kyriakidis, P., & Stannard, D. (2011). *Clinical wisdom and interventions in acute and critical care: A thinking-in-action approach* (2nd ed.). New York: Springer.

Bluvol, A., & Ford-Gilboe, M. (2004). Hope, health work and quality of life in families of stroke survivors. *Journal of Advanced Nursing, 48*(4), 322–332.

Bronfenbrenner, U. (1979). *The ecology of human development: Experiments by nature and design.* Cambridge: Harvard University Press.

Browne, G., Birch, S., & Thabane, L. (2012). *Better care: An analysis of nursing and healthcare system outcomes.* Ottawa/Toronto: Canadian Nurse/Canadian Health Services Research Foundation.

Cassidy, J., & Shaver, P. R. (2008). *Handbook on attachment* (2nd ed.). New York: Guilford Press.

Cowling, W. R. (2000). Healing as appreciating wholeness. *Advances in Nursing Science, 22*(3), 16–32.

Cozolino, L. (2013). *The social neuroscience of education: Optimizing attachment & learning in the classroom.* New York: Norton.

Deci, E. L., & Ryan, R. M. (1985). *Intrinsic motivation and self-determination in human behavior.* New York: Plenum.

Ezer, H., Bray, C., & Gros, C. P. (1997). Families' description of the nursing intervention in a randomized control trial. In L. N. Gottlieb & H. Ezer (Eds.), *A perspective on health, family, learning, and collaborative nursing: A collection of writings on the McGill model of nursing* (pp. 371–376). Montreal, CA: McGill University School of Nursing.

Ford-Gilboe, M. (2000). Dispelling myths and creating opportunity: A comparison of the strengths of single-parent and two-parent families. *Advances in Nursing Science, 23*(1), 41–58.

Gibson, C. H. (1991). A concept analysis of empowerment. *Journal of Advanced Nursing, 16*(3), 354–361.

Gottlieb, L. N. (2013). *Strengths-based nursing care: Health and healing for person and family.* New York: Springer.

Gottlieb, L. N. (2014). Strengths-based nursing: A value driven approach to health and healing. *American Journal of Nursing, 114*(8), 24–32.

Gottlieb, L. N., & Benner, P. (2013). Moving beyond deficits in nursing practice and nursing education. *Educating Nurses Newsletter*, doi: Users/ldi/Desktop/SBN.articles.2013-2014/ EducatingNursesNewsletter/Strengths-BasedNursing:MovingBeyondDeficitsinNursingP racticeandNursingEducation-Faculty.html

Gottlieb, L. N., & Feeley, N., with Dalton, C. (2006). *The collaborative partnership approach to care: A delicate balance.* Toronto: Elsevier-Mosby.

Gottlieb, L. N., & Gottlieb, B. (1998). Evolutionary principles can guide nursing's future development. *Journal of Advanced Nursing, 28*(5), 1099–1105.

Gottlieb, L. N., & Gottlieb, B. (2007). The developmental/health framework within the McGill model of nursing: "Laws of nature" guiding whole person care. *Advances in Nursing Science, 30*(1), E43–E57.

Gottlieb, L. N., & Gottlieb, B. (2013). *Strengths-based teaching and learning: An instructor's manual.* New York: Springer.

Gottlieb, L. N., Gottlieb, B., & Shamian, J. (2012). Principles of strengths-based nursing leadership for strengths-based nursing care: A new paradigm for nursing and healthcare for the 21st century. *Journal of Nursing Leadership, 25*(2), 35–46.

Gottlieb, L. N., & Rowat, K. (1987). The McGill model of nursing: A practice-derived model. *Advances in Nursing Science, 9*(4), 51–61.

Harris, J. R. (2006). *No two alike: Human nature and human individuality*. New York: W. W. Norton.

Lanius, R. A., Bluhm, R. L., & Frewen, P. A. (2011). How understanding the neurobiology of complex post-traumatic stress disorder can inform clinical practice: A social cognitive and affective neuroscience approach. *Acta Psychiatrica Scandinavica, 124*, 331–348.

Lieberman, M. D. (2013). *Social: Why our brains are wired to connect*. New York: Crown.

Lopez, S. J., & Snyder, C. R. (Eds.). (2011). *Oxford handbook of positive psychology*. New York: Oxford University Press.

McAllister, M. (2003). Doing practice differently: Solution-focused nursing. *Journal of Advanced Nursing, 41*(6), 528–535.

Miller, W. R., & Rollnick, S. (2002). *Motivational interviewing: Preparing people for change* (2nd ed.). New York: Guilford Press.

Morgan, S. & Yoder, L.H. (2012). A concept-analysis of person-centered care. *Journal of Holistic Nursing, 30*(1), 6–15.

Newman, M. A. (2008). *Transforming presence: The difference that nursing makes*. Philadelphia: F. A. Davis.

Nightingale, F. (1860). *Notes on nursing: What it is and what it is not*. London, UK: Harrison.

Pless, I. B., Feeley, N., Gottlieb, L. N., Rowat, K., Dougherty, G., & Willard, B. (1994). A randomized trial of a nursing intervention to promote the adjustment of children with chronic physical disorders. *Pediatrics, 94*(1), 70–75.

Rodwell, C.M. (1996). An analysis of the concept of empowerment. *Journal of Advanced Nursing, 23*, 305–313.

Rogers, M. E. (1970). *An introduction to the theoretical basis of nursing*. Philadelphia: F. A. Davis.

Siegel, D. J. (2012). *The developing mind: Toward a neurobiology of interpersonal experience* (2nd ed.). New York: Guilford Press.

Snyder, C. R., & Lopez, S. J. (Eds.). (2009). *Handbook of positive psychology*. New York: Oxford University Press.

Steele, S. M., & Harmon, V. M. (1979). *Value clarification in nursing*. New York: Appleton-Century-Crofts.

Schweitzer, M., Gilpin, L., & Frampton, S. (2004). Healing spaces: Elements of environmental design that make an impact on health. *Journal of Alternative and Complementary Medicine, 10*, S71–S83.

Thiots, P. A. (2011). Mechanisms linking social ties and support to physical and mental health. *Journal of Health and Social Behavior, 52*, 145–161.

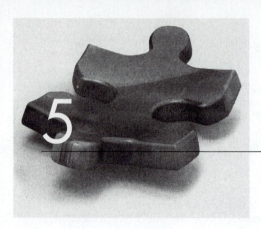

Ireland: The Model of Personhood

Geraldine McCarthy and Margaret Landers

INTRODUCTION

The philosophy underpinning the Irish nursing model of personhood is humanism. The concept of caring is fundamental to nurses' understanding of human nature. The earliest theoretical framework for nursing and midwifery in Ireland was based on the medical model (Cassels, 1908). Over time, knowledge was augmented by focusing on the care of patients with certain medical or surgical conditions. In the period from 1970 to 1980, nursing predominantly adapted the theoretical perspectives of either Henderson (1969) or Roper, Logan, and Tierney (1983), the latter a predominantly needs-based model. During the historical evolution of the profession and under the influence of Florence Nightingale, the religious orders who held prominent positions within the Irish health care system, and the cultural influences ensured that Irish nurses were introduced to spiritual and holistic concepts. Nurses are recruited from a predominantly Celtic society (Clearly & Connolly, 2005). There has never been a shortage of applicants for nursing. The perceived need for a model that reflects the focus of nursing within an Irish cultural perspective led to the development of the model of personhood.

Background

The model of personhood was first published in 2010 in the article "A Conceptual Model of Nursing: A Model of Personhood for Irish Nursing" (McCarthy and Landers, 2010). The motivation for the model's development originated from the authors' desire to present a conceptualization of the core values of nursing in an Irish society. These core values are predominantly influenced by Celtic society, Irish language, Irish customs, and the Catholic religion.

Key Concepts of the Model

The core concepts of the model are presented bilingually (McCarthy and Landers, 2010). They provide a basis for nursing practice in an Irish context. Key concepts are person, health, environment, and nursing. Core concepts of the person are *anam cara* (soul friend), *spioraid* (spirit), *aire* (caring), *gra* (love), and *dochas* (hope).

RELATIONSHIP TO CONCEPTS INHERENT IN THE METAPARADIGM OF NURSING

Nursing is a sensing process whose focus is the person and her or his unique situation. Nursing is concerned with the physical, psychological, emotional, sociological, and spiritual dimensions requiring care but in the context of a philosophy, which gives value to the concept of *personhood*. This gives credence to a person's ability to conceptualize herself or himself as being a person with moral, psychological, and cognitive dimensions that are acknowledged by significant others as being unique to that individual. The perspective requires the person to be self-aware and to watch over "the self" by changing life situations (such as illness and infirmity) or along the continuum from health to illness and youth to aged. In this way, nursing is individualized and based on care required to meet particular needs. The involvement of the person and family is also vital. A nurse uses all of the senses in the process of nursing. In familiar and unfamiliar situations, all of the senses are alerted: the eye (to see), the ear (to hear), touch (to feel and communicate), and self (as presence). Traditionally, the eyes are "said to be the windows of the soul," and the "soul writes the story of its life in the contours of the face" (Donoghue, 1999, 88). Nurses know and understand the meaning of this first statement. The eye is selective in what it sees. It is rarely judgmental but assessing and communicating in nature. Nurses select what to see through their own personal experience and self-knowledge. Criteria can be professional, but more important ones are personal with attributes developed through nature and nurture. The eyes of nurses can see pain, hurt, truth, avoidance, distrust, doubt, and love.

The tongue is the organ of speech. Words are an expression of a person's physical, emotional, and spiritual dimensions. Nurses communicate continually with multiple patients and the manner and tone of the words used are of great importance. To those in distress, soft words spoken can convey an openness to "The I-Thou relationships" as described by Martin Buber (2000). Harsh words convey impatience, disinterest, and a dismissive response. Contemporary literature applauds silence and reflection. The achievement of confidence in silence is a tenet of most ancient cultures, and the development of this attribute in the nurse is vital. In the silence of the night, patients often speak the "unspoken," and the nurse must respond appropriately. Linked to speech is the sense of hearing. Compassionate listening that can bring the nurse in touch with both what is said and unsaid is important. Touch connects people in a very intimate manner. Nurses use their hands constantly. Touch can confirm the presence of another and can comfort, sooth, and express feelings such as tenderness or reassurance. Touch can foster warmth and reassurance. It is the sense through which people experience pain and can be used to heal.

Presence is the manner in which we meet another person. Donoghue (1999, 173) says that "presence is the soul texture of the person." Presence creates atmosphere and can be positive and therapeutic. Nurses by their presence and use of the attributes just detailed can create and enhance the nurse–patient relationship and create an atmosphere conductive to health and healing.

Definition and Description of Person(s)

A *person* is a unique human being. In the model of personhood, both the person requiring or receiving nursing care (the patient) and the nurse are considered unique persons comprising spiritual, biological, emotional, and sociological dimensions. Each part works in harmony with the whole. The biological dimension is a person's "house of belonging" in this world. The emotional dimension is an inherent dimension that, in health, acts in concert with the biological and spiritual dimensions. The spiritual is the soul; it surrounds the body, is not just within it. That the human body as an expression of the soul is explicably illustrated in the mythical Irish story of the Children of Lir who were turned into Swans (yet retaining their human-ness) by their jealous stepmother. They remained as swans for 900 years until Christianity came to Ireland. The soul's light may be brought into the body through prayer, meditation, and reflection. These human dimensions are in constant dynamic interaction.

Definition and Description of Environment

In the model, *environment* takes account of the context in which nursing care is given. It emphasizes the need to consider the environment in which the patient is nursed in promoting optimum return to health. A differentiation is made between the internal and external environment in which nursing care is given. The patient may be nursed in a hospital where organizational and professional diversity and cultural perspectives differ. They patient can also be cared for in the home context that can involve other persons from young to old and different economic and social situations. Trust and respect for the person within the environment of care form the basis of a person-hood approach to practice. The model shows a bidirectional relationship between the core characteristics of the person as mentioned earlier: aire (caring); gra (love), docas (hope), spioraid (spirit), and the environment. It proposes that each nurse recognizes the therapeutic effect of a profes-sional caring (aire) environment for people who are ill. In the health care context, the nurse encounters many situations and perspectives that pro-vide wider understandings for viewing the person within the context of the environment.

Definition and Description of Health

The model of personhood acknowledges that individuals live out their lives in accordance with their own beliefs and values of what constitutes health and well-being. *Health* is equated with the ability to function as an independent individual in society. Conversely, a deficit in health status reduces the ability to be fully independent. Therefore, the goal of nursing is to enable each person to achieve an optimum level of health and independence. The nurse, the patient, and the family mutually agree to the goals of the care plan. The realization of goals requires commitment from the person but also requires the nurse's skills and knowledge. Healing is an important outcome and is supported through individually focused nursing care that considers the immediate health care need. Healing is done in the context of a philosophy that takes account of the full meaning of the concept *personhood*. Similar to other conceptual frameworks, health is considered as a continuum from illness to health. It includes the person's own sense of wellness.

RELATIONSHIP AMONG THE MODEL'S CONCEPTS AND COMPONENTS

All elements of the model are affected when individuals encounter illness, but one may be the primary focus. Based on the Irish Celtic cul-tural perspective, persons have the characteristics of caring, love, hope, and spirit. These dimensions together combine to merge into a concept called *personhood*. The model includes interrelationships between con-cepts central to nursing. Figure 5–1 represents the model of personhood diagrammatically in a circle. The circle is an old and powerful symbol; the world, sun, and moon are circles; day and night and the tides follow a circular motion, stones are in circles, and forts and watchtowers in Ireland were build in a circular form. The innermost circle contains the person as a unique individual in health or in ill health, surrounded by the anam care (soul friend) who provides care through a sensing process. The outside circle represents the environment within which care is given and is seen as cyclical from home to hospital with halfway houses, community hospitals, nursing homes, and other facilities also available.

Anam is the Gaelic for *soul*, and *cara* is the word for *friend*. In the early Celtic church, a person who acted as teacher, companion, and spiritual guide and to whom another person revealed hidden thoughts and shared the innermost self was the *anam cara*. The relationship that developed was an act of recognition: The friend of the person's soul joined the person in a spiritual trusting relationship that transcends Christianity. In the model of personhood, the nurse is the *anam cara* of each patient nursed. Similar views were reflected in the works of earlier nurse theorists. The Peplau (1952) were the first theorists who articulated the significance of establishing a helping trusting relationship with the person as a basis for the delivery of therapeutic care. Henderson (1991) defined nursing in functional terms. She advocated for an emphatic understanding of individual needs by "getting inside the skin" of each patient.

Spioraid **(Spirit).** Spiritual care has been an integral element of nursing care for decades (Costello, Atinaja-Faller, & Hedberg, 2012). The concept is complex and involves religious beliefs, hope, and moral values such as respect for persons. The concept of spirituality has been a major influence in Irish history and is today an important force in the day-to-day lives of people. This is demonstrated through the playing of the angelus on national radio and television at noon and 6 PM each day. Although the concepts of religion (belief in a God) and spirituality (the quest to find meaning) can have different meanings to people, there is a common belief that they are intertwined, and the terms are used interchangeably in the Irish context. In fact, when referring to the concept *spioraid* (spirit), Larkin (1998) writes of nurses' belief in an "existential being" and cherished religious convictions that exist in relation to death and dying. Spirituality allows people to transcend the helplessness of a situation and provides some hope and meaning in life, even though they have a life-threatening illness. *Spirit* also is used to describe one's zest for life, one's intangible presence, or that which leaves the body when one dies to enter the spirit world.

Aire **(Caring).** Caring and nursing have always been thought of synonymously. Caring as a central concept has led to the development of a number of international caring theories including the theory of human caring (Watson, 1988) and the theory of transcultural caring (Leininger, 1991). The significance of the concept *caring* for the discipline of nursing has been identified in Celtic and Irish nursing literature. Health care has historically been defined from a paternalistic perspective and the traditional biomedical science models. However, from an Irish perspective, it is defined as maternalistic and holistic; most nurses today in Ireland are women. Caring is an integral component of nursing. The term *soul friend*, or *anam chara*, describes the caring presence of the nurse. The central focus of the concept relates to the sensitivity required in accepting and understanding peoples' views of health, illness, dying, and living. It also involves being sincere and open in regard to the choices available to people. An unconditioned positive regard for another is necessary to truly connect with that person. Making people aware of the options available to them positions to them choose more freely among alternatives without feeling alone.

    Gra (Love).   *Gra* is the Irish word for *love* and has not always been explicitly expressed in Irish life but has been implicit as Eames wrote "I enjoyed the happiest of childhoods in a home where love did not have to be spoken—it was there all of the time, unspoken at times, but apart of the air we breathed" (Kearney 1997, 48). Love begins by exhibiting warmth and paying attention to another. Paul's letter to the Corinthians (New Jerusalem Bible, Chapter 13) states that "love is always patient and kind; it is never boastful or conceited; it is never rude or selfish; it does not take offence. Love is always ready to excuse, to trust, to hope and to endure whatever comes." Larkin's (1998) study referred to respondents' use of the word *gramhar* (*loving*) to describe the shared knowledge that exists between nurses and their patients in relation to death and dying. The term signifies the sense of togetherness and community spirit that exits between Irish people at a time of loss. This is seen in particularly in Ireland when "wakes" are still commonly held at times of death (often in the person's home); neighbors and friends comfort mourners; and in villages and towns, businesses are closed as a sign of mourning and respect for family members' grief. Mass cards are commonly sent for the dead, and it is traditional for the family to receive hundreds of sympathy letters and cards from friends and acquaintances. Fitzgerald and van Hooft (2000) concluded that a distinct difference exists between the concepts *aire* and *gramhar* when discussed in the context of nursing practice. *Gramhar* is demonstrated in practice when the nurse provides unselfish care that goes beyond caring for the self without reciprocity. This description of "loving" can be compared to the concept of *disinterested love* illustrated in "the careful nursing system." The term *disinterested love*, identified by Catherine

McAuley, also implies that the nurse operates from an altruistic position and provides care for each person without seeking personal gain (Meehan, 2003).

Presencing is a central concept in Parse's (1987) theory of human becoming. Parse's view is founded on existential phenomenology and requires the nurse to be "truly present with the person" in order to come to know what is important for the person in regard to his or her health and well-being. Love can be expressed in presencing (i.e., being with) and for a person who is in need of care; the presence of the nurse can provide comfort and humanity. In today's health care system, presence is sometimes absent in acute care units but always present in critical situations (one sees a number of people sitting outside intensive care units), hospice care, and in the home. The lack of presence in some situations results from contextual factors, but the concept should be held close to the nurse's activity.

Dochas (Hope).   Lohne and Severinsson (2006) identified a link between hope and spirituality in their research findings that "the power of hope: patients' experiences of hope a year after acute spinal cord injury" and that "the power of hope" had two subthemes: "will, faith and hope" and "hoping, struggling and growing." The power of hope was interpreted as the individual having experienced the meaning a year after the injury, mainly expressed through will power. Thus, hope is a multifactorial, complex feeling present at different times throughout life. It springs the eternal in the human, is held in the heart, and is often the imperceptible dimension that keeps the spirit alive when a person encounters health or other challenges. Faith in God is part of the Irish culture and of hope. Meditation, prayers, and pilgrimages to holy places in search of a miracle remain common religious practices within Irish culture. Hope is enhanced and supported by good interpersonal relationships and shared values and beliefs. It is linked to senses and can be observed in the eyes and articulated in the voice. The individual beliefs of the person and the meaningfulness of those beliefs are manifest in the hope that they express. In practice, the power of hope is influenced by the meaning and significance that patients ascribe to their illness.

CONCLUSION

This chapter presents a model of personhood influenced by a predominantly Celtic society, Irish language, Irish customs, and the Catholic religion. The key concepts addressed are person, health, environment and nursing. Central concepts relating to the person and to nursing itself within the model are *anam cara*, *spioraid*, *aire*, *gra*, and *dochas*. Nursing is presented as a sensing process with emphasis on seeing, hearing, touching, and presencing.

REFERENCES

Buber, M. (2000). *I and thou*. (R. Gregor-Smith, Trans.). New York: Scribner Classics. (Original work published 1958).

Cassels, H. (1908). *Science and art of nursing*. London: Waverly.

Cleary, J., & Connolly, C. (Eds.). (2005). *Modern Irish culture*. Cambridge: University Press.

Connell Meehan, T. (2003). Careful nursing: A model for contemporary nursing practice. *Journal of Advanced Nursing, 44*(1), 99–107.

Costello, M., Atinaja-Faller, J., & Hedberg, M. (2012). The use of simulation to instruct students on the provision of spiritual care: A pilot study. *Journal of Holistic Nursing,* 277–281.

Donoghue, J. (1999). *Anan Cara—Spiritual wisdom from the Celtic world*. London: Bantam.

Fitzgerald, F., & van Hooft, S. (2000). A Socratic dialogue on the question 'what is love in nursing'? *Nursing Ethics, 7*, 481–491.

Henderson, V. (1969). *Basic principles of nursing care*. Geneva: International Council of Nurses.

Henderson, V. (1991). *The Nature of nursing: Reflections after 25 years*. New York: National League for Nursing.

Kearney, R. (1997). *Postnationalist Ireland—Politics, culture, philosophy*. London: Routledge.

Larkin, P. (1998) The lived experience of Irish palliative care nurses. *International Journal of Palliative Care, 4*(3), 120–126.

Leininger, M. M. (1991). *Culture care diversity and universality: A theory of nursing*. New York: National League of Nursing Press.

Lohne, V., & Severinsson, E. (2006). The power of hope: Patients' experiences of hope a year after acute spinal cord injury. *Journal of Clinical Nursing, 15*, 315–323.

McCarthy, G., & Landers, M. (2010). A conceptual model of nursing: A model of personhood for Irish nursing. *Nursing Science Quarterly, 123*(4), 343–347.

Meehan T.C. (2003) Careful nursing: a model for contemporary nursing practice. *Journal of Advanced Nursing, 44*, 99–107.

Parse, R. R. (1987). *Nursing science: Major paradigms, theories, and critiques*. Philadelphia: Saunders.

Peplau, H.E. Peplau, H.E.(1952). *Interpersonal relations in nursing*. New York: Putman.

Roper, N., Logan, M., & Tierney, A. (1983, March). A model of nursing. *Nursing Times, 2*.

Watson, J. (1988). *Nursing: Human science and human care, a theory of nursing*. New York: National League for Nursing.

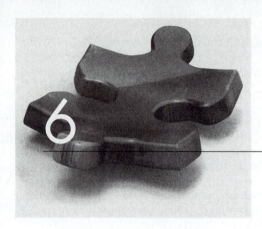

6

Italy: Nursing as a Stimulus of Health-Harmony

Renzo Zanotti

INTRODUCTION: BASIC ELEMENTS OF THE NURSING AS STIMULUS OF HEALTH-HARMONY MODEL

The *nursing as stimulus of health-harmony* model draws inspiration from the organismic approach of general system theory (von Bertalanffy, 1968), specifically regarding the conceptualization of self-regulating and feedback processes; from Prigogine (Prigogine & Stengers, 1999) on energy dissipation processes; from Kelly's (1963) theory of personal constructs to connect the biological with the cognitive domain and the behavior with perception and prediction. Also Rogers' (1970) understandings of the dynamics of energy for health and Henderson's (1966) definitions of independence in health were useful when linking the concepts of the organism and health with the concept of nursing.

Essentially, the nursing as stimulus of health-harmony model interprets the human being as an organism (a living system) with great capacity for self-regulation and for generating meanings and expectations. An organism is healthy when it can control any changes in the intensity of its processes and keep them in harmony whereas loss of control coincides with disease.

Professional nursing stimulates people to retain or regain control over process changes through prevention, compensation, or rehabilitation mechanisms that the people can activate or mediate with their behavior. Unlike medicine, nursing lacks the power to obtain a direct effect on a person's processes; instead, nursing helps to modify those effects in a given context and interpret and predict them so that people can themselves modulate the intensity of processes or outputs. Nursing is effective through modifications that are not biological but functional and behavioral and on the plane of awareness.

These factors mean that two conditions are necessary for the non-medical practice of professional nursing: patients (a) play an active part and (b) have the potential capacity to care for themselves independently. The socially acknowledged role of professional nursing does not have the power to decide and implement direct effects on the biological and functional structures of patients in the nurse's care. This power lies with pharmacological medicine and surgery (the fact that nurses may be qualified to undertake certain medical activities does not make these activities "nursing" because they still belong to the sphere of medicine). The real power of nursing lies in stimulating patients to gain better control over their own processes. In this sense, nursing stimulates the development of an increased harmony in the psychophysical processes that identify an individual's state of health.

PARADIGM OF THE MODEL OF NURSING AS STIMULUS OF HEALTH-HARMONY

The concepts of person, health, nursing, and environment in relationship with the model are defined in the following sections.

Person

A *person* is a dynamic system interacting with the environment and characterized by awareness of the sense of the ability to translate the reality the person perceives into subjectively meaningful symbols, relations, and models. A person actively constructs his or her reality in a continuous constructing-restructuring process. According to Kelly (1963), direct contact with the perceived reality is mediated by the person's interpretation because a person's processes are psychologically channeled by the ways in which he or she anticipates events. Therefore, a person communicates on the strength of expectations that integrate experience, sensory perception, and predictions that the person experiences and subsequently reassesses.

Persons are individuals capable (or potentially capable) of interpreting themselves and their environment, of assigning symbols and meanings, of experiencing emotions, and of adopting interactive behavior. Persons

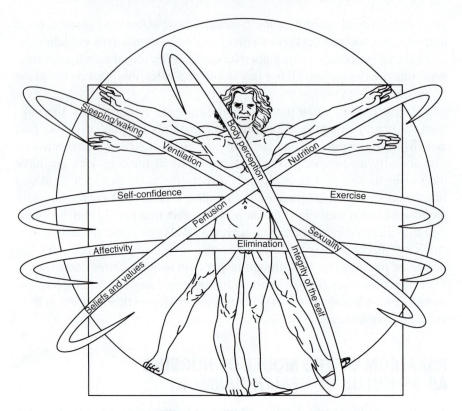

FIGURE 6–1 The Person-System.

actively construct a subjective reality into which they translate the perceived world.

   Awareness is the outcome of a systemic integration of cognitive and biological processes and products. It is an emerging quality generated by the system, not by single processes. Persons perceive the world and take action in relation to the state of their processes and to the products of their interactions; in other words, their behavior depends on their level of awareness.

Health

Health is a person's capacity to adjust the activity of her or his psychophysical processes in response to the perceived reality or to biological needs. Any process adjustment (or fluctuation) must remain within an allowable range dictated by the nature of the process (its component structures and functions) and by the system's need for its output (and the need for this output determines the importance of the process). A controlled modulation of the intensity of the system's processes ensures that their output satisfies biological and psychosocial needs. The balance achieved between needs and responses decides the system's health. The degree to which a person is able to modulate processes, or possible outputs, coincides with her or his health potential, which can also be activated and influenced by exogenous factors.

Health is a quality that emerges from the harmonious fluctuation of all the processes consistent with the organism's needs. All biological and cognitive processes have functioning dynamics that enable their output to be adapted to the system's changing physical and relational needs. *Health* is therefore a state (or quality) of a system characterized by controlled and harmonious process dynamics that serve the system's needs. An organism's capacity to control and modulate the intensity of its processes is influenced by numerous factors, including the biological integrity of its structures; its cognitive-interpretative activity, physical, and social changes in its environment; and the organism's energy reserves.

Nursing

Nursing is primarily a social activity to assist people with actions they are unable to perform unaided. Nursing becomes "professional" (and differs from "social" nursing) when the activity involved in it is competent and governed by the laws of the country concerned. A professional nurse takes action to (a) deliver medical care as part of patient care services and processes and (b) stimulate patients' health potential to help them manage their own health better. This second element defines the professional nurse as an entity separate from medicine: unlike the medical profession, nurses are not empowered to take action directly on a patient's processes; instead, they serve as external stimuli to induce the person to modulate the intensity of his or her processes or outputs. Nursing takes effect not on a biological level but on the functional plane and the patient's awareness. This means that, without the patient's active participation, the nurse's power of intervention would be limited to the role of social nursing in the sense of assisting patients in need of care.

The therapeutic potential of professional nursing has to do with the feasibility of improving patients' health according to their level of independence (exploiting their potential). Independence is a necessary condition for the quality of life of individuals, their families, and their social groups.

TABLE 6–1   Processes and Components with Specific Aspects of Nursing Interest from the Nursing as a Stimulus of Health-Harmony Theory Perspective[a]

		Processes and Components	
DIMENSION	Human Processes	Process Components	Aspects of Interest to Professional Nursing
FUNCTIONING	Metabolism	Nutrition	Ingestion of food incongruous with the organism's energy needs with observable consequences in weight/height ratio and blood chemistry
		Elimination of renal filtrate	Altered bladder emptying with consequent bladder stagnation or unwanted urine leakage
		Elimination of intestinal products	Altered intestinal emptying with consequent constipation, unwanted passage of feces, or altered emptying rhythm
	Sleeping-waking	Sleeping-waking cycle	Altered sleeping-waking cycle with consequences on performance and cognitive vigilance and perception of fatigue
	Motor capacity	Exercise	Insufficient physical activity for the purposes of preserving the functionalities of the structure/organism with consequences for the functionalities of related processes
EXCHANGE	Breathing	Ventilation	Mechanics of respiratory activity insufficient for the needs of the organism with consequent limited tolerance of physical exercise
	Blood circulation	Perfusion	Insufficient intake of nutrients and oxygen for cellular needs with immediate consequences on the state of perfused tissues and subsequently on the whole system
SELF	Self-perception	Body perception	Altered mental representation of the body's structure or parts or spatial positions of parts or all of the body
		Self-confidence	Altered self-image concerning potential, capabilities, or social sphere
		Integrity of the self	Altered sense of risk in relation to present or future events with consequent defensive reactions
		Affectivity	Inability to create, maintain, or modify significant relationships with others
		Sexuality	Incongruous perception of sexual identity and/or capacity and/or desire
	Understanding	Consistency of beliefs and values	Discrepancy between the person's cultural patterns and events that occur expressed in emotional behavior and interactions

[a] All aspects may be treated without any use of medical treatments or complementing medical treatment.
Source: R. Zanotti. (2010). "Philosophy and Theory in the Modern Conceptualization of Professional Nursing". PICCIN: Padova

Environment

Everything perceived by a person as being outside himself or herself is the environment. It generates stimuli, demands, and energy, which influence the activity of the organism's processes and needs.

The *environment* is a set of meanings constructed by individuals on the strength of their sensory activity, cognitive interpretation, and social and affective expectations (the family is an environment in which people identify themselves and are connected by meaningful relationships). For nursing, the environment also defines roles ranging from independent and exclusive to multiprofessional (at home and in hospital) and settings that can modify the professional nurse's decisions and actions depending on the resources available and the obstacles encountered.

RELATIONSHIPS AMONG CONCEPTS

The conceptual structure of the nursing as stimulus of health-harmony model relies on four main relationships.

1. A person is a psychophysical organism consisting of parts and processes; the concept interprets itself and the environment, generates meanings and expectations, and interacts with physical and social surroundings.
2. A person's health depends on the level of his or her control over the activity of his or her processes.
3. Environmental stimuli and a person's expectations influence the activity of his or her processes, the variability of which must remain within an allowable range depending on the energy available, the nature of the structures generating the process, and the specific control system involved.
4. Expressed health is the condition deriving from a controlled adjustment of all the processes within their allowable range of variation so that the needs and output, energy available, and energy consumption are congruous.

The health potential of an organism is a condition so that it can further modulate the activity of a process beyond its normally allowable limit without losing control in order to supply a peak output in conditions of exceptional request. Health potential is the extent of this capacity for further intensity of processes' variation and serves as a reserve that can be used by the organism to increase specific performances.

Consequently, an organism's overall health depends on the capacity to control the variations of its processes in order to face the requests. The ability to maintain control over changes in processes fluctuations is also an expression of flexibility, or an organism's adaptability to cope with changes in the internal or external environment.

Disease

Disease occurs when an organism loses control over the activity of one or more processes and is consequently unable to maintain a balance between request and process output. Disease involves a lower or higher process output and energy consumption inconsistent with the organism's needs, which gradually disrupts other related structures and processes, leading to an ever-greater loss of harmony between the processes and the system's needs.

The system's loss of control that lies behind the pattern of disease demands action from outside the system even without active participation of the individual involved, and this action sets the stage for that patient's cure. In its proper medical sense, *cure* is an independent capacity to modify an organism's biology to neutralize harmful substances, repair disruptions, and replace parts. Cure is necessary every time the loss of control over a process cannot be accomplished by remodulating other processes or with functional adjustments (as in chronic disease). Therefore, the system change is not disease, but a temporary disruption, that can be brought under control by temporary exogenous stimulation leading to process readjustments of which the organism is still capable.

Local or systemic reactive patterns within the organism's health potential are phenomena of interest for nursing research and activity of care. Professional nursing always takes action to stimulate better tuning of processes and coping within the organism's behaviors to prevent disharmony, probability of disease, or further disruptive consequences. Professional nursing seeks to activate a person's health potential when his or her capacity to control one or more processes is limited as the result of biological or cognitive factors or influences.

In care activity, professional nursing functions as a stimulus for a person's process and activities. Thus, nursing requires, at least to some degree, a person's active participation to enhance his or her range of control. Helping people to better tune into their processes, nursing functions as a stimulus of harmony and allows for better health of their organism.

ANALYSIS AND EVALUATION: RELATIONSHIP AMONG THE MODEL'S CONCEPTS AND COMPONENTS

Nature of the Process

A *process* is a sequence of orderly actions taken by correlated biological or functional structures (physical or cognitive behavior) to generate an output. Process dynamics are essential to life. The sequential activity of a process enables single components (organs, cells, or apparatuses) to operate periodically according to the biological demands of the cellular processes. The concept of process is equally applicable to cognitive activity (self-confidence, affectivity, etc.) if it is depicted as phases of perception, interpretation, and prediction arranged sequentially into a process. Processes always function periodically or cyclically, as in sleeping-waking for instance, or breathing, blood circulation, and so on, according to the system's organization.

Stimuli and Process Activities

Every process in a person–organism is managed by control systems based on feedbacks in order to maintain consistency between the output of the processes and the requests of the organisms. If the system demands that a specific output be minimal, that process will tend to diminish in intensity to a minimal level within its allowable range of variation in accordance with the system's requirements. Deep relaxation, meditation, and non-REM sleep are exemplary situations in which the system's requests are low and the intensity of various processes is consequently minimal.

Energy for Process Activity

Life is continuous activity, endless movement; as a process, life is a product and expression of dynamics, which involves the use and transformation of energy. Therefore, the system's dynamism (its health) relies on the availability and effective use of energy. The sequential activity of a process makes it effective to control the use of energy by component structures (organs, cells, or apparatuses) because they operate at a different intensity when energy is needed for a given process phase involving the structures. Every process needs energy for its activity. There are various forms of energy to suit the nature of a process's components: For instance, the blood circulation process exploits pressure gradients produced by muscle and biochemical dynamics whereas self-confidence requires confirmation and gratification. The nature of the energy depends on the nature of the process it supplies. Two conditions should be considered:

1. The availability of specific energy is a necessary condition for the adaptive oscillation of a process to be activated.
2. The specific energy must be available in sufficient quantity for a process to oscillate with an intensity that meets the system's needs. So, the system must use mechanisms that provide information on the level of energy available for adaptive purposes.

Process Variations with a Compensatory Function

An organism's system has the capacity to adjust a process in relation to the type and intensity of a stress and to the quantity of output the system needs. A process is controlled with specific adaptive sectorial variations (e.g., vasoconstriction in the extremities) in the various phases of the process. When an equilibrium is reached, the process is restored to its normal intensity. If a system's capacity for process control is inadequate, it will modify its overall balance by adjusting several processes with a compensatory intent in an effort to preserve maximal harmony between its processes.

The activity of every process correlates with all other processes. For instance, a foot's sensitivity may be insufficient if the local blood circulation is inadequate; in coma, altered cognitive processes prevent the system's functional response to pressure on the tissues (decubitus).

If, even after adjusting its intensity, the process still fails to produce the necessary output, this discrepancy will stimulate changes of intensity in other processes, disrupting the system's balance. Depending on the type and intensity of a process's stimulation and/or alteration, the system takes increasingly intense compensatory action to restore the process to its normal intensity and stabilize the system. It is in this sense that we can understand such manifestations as boredom, delirium, and dreaming, which reflect the organism's capacity to stimulate cognitive and biological processes. The system's adaptability and consequent health potential coincide with a range determined by the organism's capacity to control the variability of its processes.

A process thus has a given range of variability that the system can use for the purposes of its adaptability (or health potential). For instance, the system can tolerate marked changes in its respiratory process during intense physical activity, providing its circulatory and metabolic processes as well as its bodily perception and self-confidence are adequate. If not, the outcome could be dyspnea or muscle cramps and a sense of inadequacy and panic.

Signs of Inadequate Process Control

The organic system compensates for incongruous process variations that are not functional to its output request by modulating other processes; this becomes manifest in "nonspecific" behavior associated with the "specific" behavior generated by the incongruous process. The pattern of empirically detectable specific and nonspecific signs reveals the nature, intensity, and diffusion of the incongruity or disharmony between the processes. In a system with plenty of health potential, the discrepancy is managed by means of further variations and adaptations of the system's behavior to minimize or adapt to the discrepancy.

Incongruous process changes that occur in a system equipped with health potential create a condition of interest for care provision because the incongruity can be reduced or eliminated by providing the system with the elements it lacks or by stimulating more effective compensatory behavior (training for self-care) to control its process variations.

Judging Incapacity as a Nursing Diagnosis

The onset of an inadequate control over process variations is identifiable from physiological and behavioral signs that partly reveal variations in process intensity (erythema is evidence of an increased local blood flow) and partly indicate the system's adaptive responses to such variations (e.g., an increased local sensitivity to the touch). A set of changes forms a pattern expressing the nature of the disrupted process and the level of the system's involvement. Searching for this pattern, starting from elementary signs of change, provides a semiotic frame leading to the identification of the causal process and the severity of the disruption (elements of the diagnostic judgment). It follows that, in order to derive coherent activities, a diagnosis must describe three dimensions:

1. The altered process, which emerges from patterns of behavior described using defining names.
2. The level of difference from the individual's baseline expressed using process or output variation qualifiers.
3. One or more elements identified as the likely cause of the variation (if any).

Ascertaining Health Potential

When a process discrepancy is identified, the person's health potential must be assessed. A condition warranting professional nursing coincides with a clinical judgment of "inadequate control/compensation" for specific processes in a given patient (diagnosis). The diagnosis must be correlated with the patient's chances of improvement (capacity–objective) achievable with nursing measures.

Change as Disease

Disease is an expression of disharmony beyond the system's control and is characterized by the system's inability to reduce the discrepancy between processes' outcomes and the organism's request to an acceptable level or to compensate with the system's behaviors (lack of health potential). Disease requires external modifying interventions (medical cure).

RELATIONSHIP OF THEORY TO NURSING AND HEALTH RESEARCH

Since 1989, the theory of nursing as stimulus of health-harmony (Zanotti, 1989) has been adopted for research. It includes:

1. *Assessment and evaluation systems for nursing practice:* This line of research, aimed at developing the model's semiotics, generated a set of indicators with a variable degree of specificity for identifying states of altered process control. Each alteration was attributed to a minimum system of indicators to use as signs (excluding all those potentially linked to disease). The outcome of this line of research, conducted with the participation of hundreds of nurse–observers in various Italian hospitals, led to the definition of a minimum system of empirical indicators for observing process changes of nursing interest. Based on this information, interpretative and predictive models were defined on the strength of relationships between possible causal events, alterations in parts of processes of interest to nursing, and likely empirical indicators of these alterations. All diseases and disease indicators were excluded (Zanotti, 1998).

2. *Informatic decision support systems:* This line of research enabled the relational models to be translated into mathematical models based on matrix algebra. In accordance with probability theory, the mathematical models weighted the intensity of links between the set of indicators and causes (behavior and living conditions, presence of disease, and setting) with possible process changes, providing a probabilistic estimate for nursing diagnostics and prognosis.

   The mathematical models were subsequently converted into a computer software NIMMO (Nursing Information Matrix-Modeling) marketed by SUMMA Editor (Padova) for use in clinical medicine and training (Zanotti, 1994). The line of research currently focuses on experimenting with computerized systems for predicting outcomes starting from patients' initial characteristics.

3. *Assessment scales and intervention systems:* This line of research led to the fine adjustment of two scales, ASGO 1 and 2 (functionality and competence), for assessing health potential levels in hospitalized patients. The scales were validated on tens of thousands of patients in a number of studies starting in 1994.

4. *Expert systems for predicting care commitment and possible outcome:* This line of research, which is currently underway, applies the weighted profiles derived from the ASGO and the links with the weighted intervention profiles. The output is a descriptive mathematical system for linking admission status, possible status on discharge, and type and frequency of interventions. The model is being tested in various hospitals in several Italian regions and will enable the construction of large databases that can be used for an ongoing improvement of the model of nursing as stimulus of health-harmony.

5. *Effectiveness of clinical nursing interventions:* Experimental and quasi-experimental designs have been conducted to test the feasibility and effectiveness of remodulating stimulations on a patient's processes, particularly in sleeping disorders, anxiety (Bulfone, Quattrin, Zanotti, Regattin, & Brusaferro, 2009), pain control (Zampieron & Zanotti, 2008), and delirium in hospitalized elderly (Bonaventura & Zanotti, 2007).

RELATIONSHIP OF THE THEORY TO NURSING EDUCATION

The theory has been included in nursing training programs in various schools in the Italian regions of Tuscany (since 1992) and the Veneto. In educational terms, the nursing as stimulus of health-harmony model seeks to develop nursing skills on three levels:

1. Technology based on protocols and guidelines with no limit on the type of skill because they are all considered equivalent from the "how-to" standpoint.

2. Integrated assessment of a clinical case needing medical care, nursing, tools, and methods as well as assessment and intervention according to guidelines identified by the model.

3. Advanced nursing intervention to develop a patient's ability to control her or his process variations. On this last level, students learn more about how to plan by objectives in relation to standard guidelines, particularly in the domains of self-care for pain, stress, incontinence, and rest. The model's application is part of the official training provided at the University of Padua and at Florence University's off-campus location in Empoli.

RELATIONSHIP TO PROFESSIONAL PRACTICE

Providing care in a professional sense for people with health issues means deliberately inducing behavior to activate their health potential (if any) or, failing this, to enable new compensatory and adaptive behavior from other processes. Professional care for a person demands action designed to:

- Develop the system's capacity to control variations in its processes.
- Activate a more effective behavior in its interaction with the environment.
- Improve awareness of the self and of the environment.
- Recover the functions of one or more processes with direct (temporary) substitutive measures.

Applying the conceptuality of the nursing as stimulus of health-harmony model to clinical practice enables:

- Ascertaining a patient's health potential in relation to his or her current state of health.
- Establishing goals consistent with the activation of a patient's health potential.
- Choosing appropriate measures in terms of a patient's power and stimulatory congruence.
- Keeping the focus on the person, not only on single disorders.

The model always enables the context of the independent practice of care to be distinguishable from that of the application of care (Zanotti, 2006).

The indications on the relationships between physiological, psychic, and somatic processes provided by the model guides the practitioner toward actions, however apparently minimal, that always aim to stimulate. For instance, massage or skin friction is seen as a rhythmic stimulation of the local blood circulation to favor vasodilation and thus stimulate factors controlling the small vessels; at the same time, massaging the skin also stimulates areas of the brain (via the peripheral nerve pathways) that generate and connect proprioception as an interpretation of the body. The person treated feels a pleasant sensation on the skin that can stimulate her or his perception of physical pleasure and facilitate muscle relaxation with a feedback effect on the system that helps to reduce the person's state of anxiety. The caring action thus provides a stimulus, a factor triggering a sequence of effects on various processes and their systemic interactions.

Another example is that physical pain should always be assessed in relation to other altered processes. Pain is a subjectively interpreted stimulus connected to a process in which people fear the disrupting effects of the pain experienced as a threat to the permanence of their intact selves in the immediate future and generating anxiety (Katon, Kleinman, & Rosen, 1982). A low pain tolerance increases the expectation of pain as seen in anxious people who report experiencing more severe pain and ask for higher doses of analgesics after surgical procedures (Taenzer, Melzack, & Jeans, 1986).

The relationship between the perception of "me, here and now" and the expectations for "me, tomorrow" was also used by Pridham (1993) in a model of "internal functioning" in which pain is a process of interaction between expectations, values, beliefs, and meanings related to identity and future prospects. People who suffer from chronic pain consume energy to manage the disturbing symptom and no longer have enough energy for the dynamics of ideational and interpretative processes of the self; this frequently leads to chronic major depression. A disrupted sleeping-waking process carries a sense of chronic fatigue that influences affective and social processes, leading to isolation and solitude. An altered sleeping-waking process also means that pain is perceived as being more intense with a gradual deterioration in the harmonious relationship between the psychophysical processes and a slow destruction of the person. Meltzack and Torgerson (1971), who first investigated the existence of a relationship between the sensory perception of pain and affective processes, produced a list of adjectives for qualifying a perceived pain. The adjectives express the two domains of somatic sensations and generally negative sensations not focused on areas of the body.

If a person lacks the potential to improve control over her or his processes, nursing may offer no added benefit of improvement over and above medical care. Therefore, nursing care can assume a substitutive function and/or a medical implementing function. Care that does not pursue the stimulation of independence (in the sense of the maximal autonomy achievable for a person's quality of life, a harmony both in the interior and with the outside world as a condition for health) should be described as substitutive or basic. As such, basic care can be provided by caregivers, not professional nurses, because it does not necessitate theory but rules, procedural operations, and dedication toward the other mostly aiming to support, substitute, and provide comforting measures.

The practical application of this nursing model in hospital involves a system to ascertain a patient's process control capacity called the general assessment of hospitalized persons (ASGO) comprising two tools:

1. *ASGO 1:* A checklist for 10 functionalities that do not require medical care, each of which can be managed with supportive measures or by empowering the patient
2. *ASGO 2:* An assessment of a patient's self-care skills and knowledge for managing conditions relating to his or her functional capacities, medical care, or rehabilitation

The ASGO system is used at admission and discharge as well as every time there is a significant change in the patient's condition. Its application gives rise to a weighted "profile" that provides a qualitative and quantitative description of the patient. Profiles are grouped by type (qualitatively) and intensity (quantitatively) to decide the commitment of resources and the type of patient care path: Each type of profile corresponds to a type of care path (which is further customized). The whole system of admission-discharge assessment and care path selection has been computerized in a system for supporting nursing decision making.

This nursing model has been integrally adopted in several hospitals in Tuscany and in a hospital department in the Veneto region staffed by nurses and students (without medical staff) and dealing with a variety of cases. This hospital department also serves as an experimental laboratory for assessing the model's capacity to predict the profiles of clinical cases, the efficacy of interventions, and the long-term results after discharge. Nurses and students receive training on the model's theoretical grounds and on the use of its applications, and they operate with a computerized system for analyzing and assessing the model's capacity to interpret and predict situations, nursing interventions, and their outcomes.

REFERENCES

Bonaventura, M., & Zanotti, R. (2007). [Effectiveness of IPD treatment for delirium prevention in hospitalized elderly. A controlled randomized clinical trial]. *Professioni Infermieristiche, 60*(4), 230–236.

Bulfone T., Quattrin, R., Zanotti, R., Regattin L., & Brusaferro, S. (2009). Effectiveness of music therapy for anxiety reduction in women with breast cancer in chemotherapy treatment. *Holistic Nursing Practice, 23*(4), 238–242.

Henderson, V. (1966). *The nature of nursing: A definition and its implications for practice, research, and education.* New York: Macmillan.

Katon, W., Kleinman, A., & Rosen, G. (1982). Depression and somatization: A review. *American Journal of Medicine, 72,* 127–135.

Kelly, G. (1963). *A theory of personality: The psychology of personal constructs.* W. W. Norton.

Meltzack, R., & Torgerson, W. S. (1971). On the language of pain. *Anesthesiology, 34,* 50–59.

Pridham, K. F. (1993). Anticipatory guidance of parents of new infants: Potential contribution of the internal working model construct. *Image, 25,* 49–56.

Prigogine, I., & Stengers, I. (1999). *A new alliance. Metamorphoses of science.* Milan: Einaudi.

Rogers, M. E. (1970). *An introduction to the theoretical basis of nursing.* Philadelphia: F. A. Davis.

Taenzer, P., Meltzack, R., & Jeans, M. E. (1986). Influence of psychological factors on postoperative pain, mood and analgesic requirements. *Pain, 24,* 331–342.

von Bertalanffy, G. (1968). *General system theory: Foundations, development, applications* (rev. ed.). New York: George Braziller.

Zampieron, A., & Zanotti, R. (2008). [Pain and treatment satisfaction: An observational study]. *Professioni Infermieristiche, 61*(1), 3–8.

Zanotti, R. (1989). A model of reading needs of nursing care. *Proceedings VIII National Conference ANIARTI 11–25: Bologna.*

Zanotti, R. (1994). *NIMMO for nursing diagnoses.* Padova: SUMMA.

Zanotti, R. (1998). Caring for persons from the perspective of nursing as "stimulus of harmony-health. *Nursing World,* 1–7.

Zanotti, R. (2006). A diagnostic model for a specialist nurse. In: *Coloproctologia, Stomia e Incontinenza: Diagnosi Infermieristica e Percorsi di Assistenza,* 41–63. Roma: Carocci Faber.

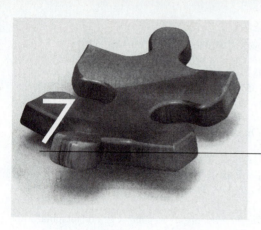

Japan: Nursing Theory of Physical Assessment

Toyoaki Yamauchi

This chapter describes Yamauchi's layered model of life function theory: the hierarchy of factors; "to live" layer, "to be alive" layer, or "able" layer, "unable" layer.

INTRODUCTION: THE NATURE OF NURSING EDUCTION IN JAPAN

Japan has two types of license for entry-level nursing practice: (a) professional nurses, who are almost equivalent to registered nurses in the United States, and (b) assistant nurses, who are similar to U.S. licensed practical nurses.

Professional nurses are educated in two-, three-, and four-year programs in nursing schools and colleges after graduation from high school. Upon passing a national examination administered by the Ministry of Health and Welfare, these professional nurses are qualified to work with doctors in hospitals and in clinics, public health centers, industry, schools, and home-visiting nurse stations.

Assistant nurses are educated in a variety of programs following junior high school. After passing a prefectural examination, they are qualified to work under the direction of doctors, dentists, and professional nurses.

Even though two levels of license for entry-level nursing practice exist, clarifying the difference in the actual working status and the scope of practice of these two types of license is difficult. In the hospital, there is often no difference in the uniform of a professional nurse and an assistant nurse and, likewise, their responsibilities can be virtually indistinguishable. In many medical facilities, most of the nursing staff are assistant nurses because of the low salaries the facilities offer. The workload and the responsibilities of professional workers are almost the same among the different license groups, but this is not reflected in the salaries or benefits between each group.

In Japan, the license and its scope of practice do not completely reflect the educational programs offered. Most professional nurses now graduate from traditional nursing schools, not from college or universities. The most serious concern raised by this type of schooling is how to clarify the characteristics in the actual daily practice based on the differences in educational backgrounds for assistant nurses versus professional nurses.

Eligibility for entrance to nursing school requires graduation from senior high school. Even though junior high school graduates are technically eligible for entrance to assistant nursing schools, most of the recently admitted students to those schools are senior high school graduates. Students who graduated from senior high school are eligible to enter a nursing school program of "assistant nurse to professional nurse" after they have three years of clinical experience. Many recent graduates from assistant nursing schools wish to enter these programs. Some assistant nurses do not take this opportunity and remain as assistant nurses because they think that there would be no actual differences in their daily practice and responsibilities after they move to the rank of professional nurses.

Rapid Growth in the Number of BSN Programs

Since 1992, the number of baccalaureate nursing programs in Japan has increased, reaching 188 in 2000. Even then, however, the total number of new nursing students enrolled in baccalaureate programs was 15,394, only 26.1% of all nursing students whereas 67.9% of new nursing students entered diploma programs. In Japan, the number of diploma programs, which are similar to those formerly prevalent in the United States, is increasing. The majority of Japan's diploma programs provide hospital-based education according to which the ideal nurse is one who strictly obeys the physician's instructions without question.

The number of four-year nursing baccalaureate programs is increasing as is the number of traditional nursing school programs. In contrast, the number of diploma schools in the United States is decreasing whereas the growth in the number of Bachelor of Science in Nursing (BSN) programs is increasing in Japan. Regional doctors' associations support the establishment and running of diploma schools for a constant output of assistant nurses to their facilities.

Education of Midwives and Public Health Nurses

Licenses for midwives and public health nurses require having a professional nurse's license. Even though the educational programs for these two licenses are provided to professional nurse licensees, the programs do not go beyond the range of undergraduate education. Entrance to neither a midwife nor a public health nurse program requires graduate education. Most four-year nursing baccalaureate programs for professional nurses provide qualified educational content for their graduates to take the examinations for a public health nurse or a midwife. Regular diploma graduates must enter additional programs to become candidates qualified to attempt these examinations after they pass the national examination for professional nurse.

Graduate Education and Clinical Studies

In addition to the increase in the number of four-year nursing baccalaureate programs in Japan, the number of graduate nursing programs is increasing. Although this growth is rapid, the total number in 2000 was small with only 127 masters' and only 61 doctoral programs in Japanese nursing education. Research and clinical studies are the main areas of focus in graduate nursing education.

In Japan, there is no one-step route to a doctorate. All doctoral students must first graduate from a master's program. Completion of these programs is required for researchers and candidates to enter doctoral programs.

Graduate educational programs focusing on clinical specialist education have been gaining in popularity recently. The Japanese Nursing Association established, and has operated, its own certification programs since 1995. Certified nurses (CNs) and certified nurse specialists (CNSs) are the two certifications. Eligibility for clinical specialists requires a minimum of a master's degree in a nursing specialty, and many graduate programs now seek to become eligible courses for candidates for the CN exam.

As the number of clinical specialist programs increases, Japan needs to provide opportunities for certified clinical specialists. In 2012, the country had 1,046 certified nurse specialists in 11 specialties and 12,522 certified nurses in 21 fields.

Nursing Staff Information for Japan

According to the country's infant mortality rate, Japan has been ranked in this category as the healthiest country surveyed. A national health status can be determined by various factors. Among them, the number of nursing staff is one of the most important indices; this number was 1,344,388

(10.540 per 1,000 population unit) in 2012, compared to 3,498,450 (11.140 per 1,000 population unit) in the United States in 2011 (OECD, 2015).

Even though the ratios of nursing staff to population in the United States and Japan are not so different, any similarity in the quality of nurses' educational background in both countries is questionable. Nursing as a profession in the United States requires higher educational preparation than in Japan, where the majority of nurses received basic nursing education through diploma programs. Until 1991, Japan had only 11 nursing baccalaureate programs in nursing whereas the United States had more than 600. In 2008, the population of Japan was 127,692,000, whereas that of the United States was 304,438,000.

YAMAUCHI'S LAYERED MODEL OF LIFE FUNCTION

This section discusses the author's theory, the *hierarchy of factors*; the "to live" layer, "to be alive" layer, or "able layer, unable layer".

Among existing nursing theories, it cannot be determined whether they are right or wrong. This depends on their organization. The basic premise common to these theories is a person leading his or her life.

Monitoring

Monitoring is an act of looking at something and is superficially regarded as a *passive activity*. However, this definition of monitoring is insufficient. For instance, it is similar to visual perception. Retinal cells respond to light coming to the eyes, and the stimulus reaches the brain's visual cortex. Unless the stimulus received by the visual cortex of the brain forms a perception, what has been seen makes no sense. What has been seen is not a reflection of a constriction of the pupils caused by dazzling lights but a consequence of responsive assessment associated with recognition of the stimulus. In other words, monitoring involves a certain degree of *assessment*, which means to understand or separate something. Assessment related to various areas ranging from emotions, such as *likes* and *dislikes*, to abstract aspects, such as *right* or *wrong*. When certain input data are given, output is generated as a result of assessment. In fact, then, monitoring is really a proactive action. Another aspect of nursing care is that monitoring items always overlap. Moreover, monitoring items regarding daily life activities can be confused because of different human systems. A new theory regarding how to monitor patients and their activities is discussed next.

According to the author's layered model of life functions, monitoring daily life activities of people is an important aspect of nursing practice, but nurses must not forget the basic premise that the human body survives as an organism. The manipulation of respiratory and circulatory functions by humans will cause great problems. These functions are designed to work regardless of the will. However, involuntary movements caused by these functions are difficult to control. In nursing care, both voluntary and involuntary movements are to be monitored. Nurses must monitor a patient's living activities and health condition to protect her or him from a life-or-death crisis. The ability to cover a broad range of patients' activities and ensure proper monitoring is essential for nursing practice so that all-encompassing care can be realized.

The author's concept of nursing is a *layered model of living functions*. In nursing practice, monitoring from both physical and lifestyle perspectives is mandatory because each interacts with the other. People live in real life, not virtual life. If the human body itself is threatened, "daily life" itself makes no sense. Nursing practice encompasses various aspects of real life: physical health where promotion of mobility is achieved, mental health where the workings of the mind are stabilized, communication where verbal contact with others occurs (at medical institutions, home, and surroundings), and a life cycle where personal timelines are reflected.

Providing Nursing Care

Nursing care works best in clinical arenas where nurses deal directly with patients. Currently, clinical practices are provided not only within medical institutions but also at various other locations.

Hospitalization is available for patients with potential risks whose health condition is not stable enough to stay at home. Physicians who have identified such risks have no choice but to advise patients to enter the hospital. So, patients are hospitalized because they need a quick response to sudden changes in their condition or have potential risks that could develop at any moment. Nurses can provide patients adequate care for daily life, but failing to find potential risks renders the activities of nurses insignificant. It is important not to overlook any possible sudden change in a patient's condition. Therefore, what is most required of nurses in clinical arenas is the ability to respond quickly to sudden changes in a patient's condition and provide appropriate care.

Prioritizing

Before anything can be prioritized, it is necessary to classify cases that require a priority access or urgent response, including, of course, a sudden change in the situation. In Japanese, the word *wakaru* (understand) is a cognate with the word *wakeru* (separate). The word *handan* (assessment) originally consists of two characters that are *han* (understand) and *dan* (separate), which implies a process of working from a chaotic state to an ordered state. Classification of something requires a policy. Without a defined policy, separating things into different categories is extremely difficult. Conversely, once a policy has been defined, how to classify its parts and the number of categories that need to be made will become easy to understand. A key to successful classification is to set a purpose. In other words, classification without any purpose is vague and realistically impossible to achieve.

To prioritize, consider the concept of *priority body*, which indicates the combined results of severity of condition, rate of change, and frequency of physical and mental aspects. When determining the priority of a patient's condition, the underlying factors considered are severity, stage of the condition, and frequency of response per unit of time. These factors are assumed not to be completely independent but interrelated. The significance of each factor varies in accordance with the original condition or circumstances.

For example, determining the priority in the case of an asthma attack depends on its frequency, severity, and the wait time until the patient receives adequate care. A comprehensive determination incorporating these factors establishes the priority. The frequency of attack can be evaluated as the number of times per month or in a semiquantitative way using a peak flow rate at the time of the attack. How often the attack occurs and how much the patient is impaired interact with each other.

The concept of prioritizing also applies to mental health. In the case of depression, mental care prioritizing involves considering factors such as its stage, its progression rate, and its incidence. Assessment seems to work well when reference to empirical knowledge is available.

Conducting Physical Assessments

Nursing practice is rooted in monitoring activities, which involve the assessment of a specific condition and are essential to nursing practice. It is important for nurses to have an assessment policy specifying the purpose for their assessment and helping them to prioritize patients for treatment. Although assessment is considered an action at a single point in time, a series of information collection and analysis should be followed before reaching assessment is completed. These processes are collectively called *assessment*. When assessment is related to physical description, it is called *physical assessment*.

Physical assessment is sometimes confused with physical examination. *Examination* refers to a means of gathering information. Nurses who have clinical experience certainly should be familiar with physical assessment. However, some may believe themselves to be less familiar with it because they misunderstand that physical assessment is the same as the examination of the full body from head to toe. Measuring blood pressure is one examination activity. For example, when the automated sphygmomanometer shows 220/120, the nurse asks how the patient feels and even urges her or him to have the value measured again. However, the automated sphygmomanometer itself simply shows the blood pressure value. A member of the medical care staff finding a person who feels dizzy should try to measure her or his blood pressure, but the automated sphygmomanometer does not wrap itself around the patient's arm without human assistance.

Knowing which patient needs blood pressure measurement and how to utilize the measured data are critical to assessment. The steps to be followed for measurement are part of an examination procedure. Nurses also perform examinations, but data collected without a clear objective or incorrectly analyzed serve no purpose.

Key to Successful Physical Assessment.

As long as a nursing action is visible, nurses can learn to perform physical assessment through training programs. However, the key to successful physical assessment is what to do before and after it. The term *physical assessment* consists of two categories, physical and assessment. The *physical* aspect involves the body, and the *assessment* is the act of judging, or evaluating, a person or situation using the data obtained for a specific purpose. Unless assessment occurs, what nurses observe or hear goes to waste.

How to Make a Physical Assessment.

Unless the points to assess are specifically defined, actual physical assessment cannot take place. For example, evaluating breath sounds requires using the sense of hearing, not of smell or touch. The fact that sound waves stimulate the acoustic sense seems from an outsider's perspective to be little different from auscultation. What differentiates sounds is attaching a significance to those heard. Thus, how nurses observe and what they are trying to find out are keys to successful assessment.

Physical assessment does not tell medical staff everything. It does not work in two instances. One is when nurses must provide much more effort than normal to achieve their goal; this is caused by a lack of training. The other is failing in an attempt at assessment caused by human limitations despite providing best efforts.

Dwelling on what went wrong in a physical assessment leads to no progress.

Being Able/Unable to Assess, Have to/Do Not Have to Assess.   To improve physical assessment, nurses need to perceive what they can and cannot do. That is, they need to recognize what must be done and what must *not* be done. Nurses are prone to trying everything in attempting to feel better after failure. Everything a nurse tries for this reason or leaves unfinished will almost certainly be completely useless. So, when a nurse thinks, "I don't have to do this," it would be more appropriate to think, "It is better not to do this."

The Pareto principle, also known as the *80–20 rule*, states that, for many events, roughly 80% of the effects come from 20% of the causes. In the 19th century, Italian economist Pareto developed the principle that 80% of sales come from 20% of clients. This principle applies not only to activities in business but also to other fields. A medical accident is no exception to this rule. For example, in the case of injection-associated accidents, it can be said that 80% of them come from 20% of the steps if the injection procedure has 10 steps. This indicates that problems do not occur at each step at the same level of frequency. So, to avoid accidents, nurses should look over an entire procedure, find out on which steps problems occur, and then deal with the steps concerned so that 80% of the accidents can be prevented. It is important to strike a proper balance between where efforts are and are not needed.

Striking a proper balance of energy use is an efficient way to prevent using efforts in vain. According to the layered model of life function theory, "doing" rather than "not doing" makes nurses feel better. Those who try to use all of their strength for every step cannot focus on the critical factors. If they recognize which item is critical and which is less critical, they can focus on the critical ones and trace a quick path through less critical ones. This principle also applies to the monitoring process. Nurses can find an assessment clue from a patient's symptoms to achieve a proper balance.

Being Accountable

The highest priority for nurses is sharing what they know with others. This is often not performed clearly in clinical practice. The key to sharing is *the ability to communicate properly*. Nursing professionals do not merely practice their skills; they must also be accountable for what they do. They need to have the ability to communicate in a persuasive manner with patients who pay money for nursing care.

Consider, for example, that one morning a nurse goes to clean a patient then decides that it is better to cancel the patient's bathing that day. The nurse made this assessment decision based on the results of monitoring. However, a nurse who fails to explain why the patient's bathing has been canceled appears not to have accepted accountability for his or her activities as a professional, even though the decision could be correct. So, nurses always must be prepared to explain their actions. They will learn how this works through on-site experience. Moreover, they may need to spend some time learning how to explain respectfully and thoroughly. Just knowing is not enough; getting others to understand is necessary.

Using the Theory for Nursing Education

This layered model of life function theory has become widely used as a basis for nursing education in Japan. Educational programs for physical assessment based on this theory include basic and introductory nursing courses, continuing courses for nursing school graduates, certified nurse courses, and even graduate school curricula. As a result, the theory is applied extensively in practical settings. In the academic domain, researchers have reported on the development of educational programs based on this theory and the measurement of their outcomes. A protocol of home-visit nursing care using this theory has been developed and put into practice, and the results have been verified as this theory being effective through studies. Considering these facts, there can be no doubt that in the fields of nursing education, nursing practice, and nursing research, the use of the layered model of life function theory will become increasingly prevalent in the future.

Textbooks and educational DVD video programs based on this author's theory of layered model of life functions are in wide circulation, having exceeded 150,000. Physical assessment based on this theory is taught widely, and as a result, is applied extensively in practice settings. Its program of physical assessment is being provided at many educational institutions at both introductory and advanced levels for continuing education of graduate and specialized nurses. In addition, the theory is applicable not only to clinical practice in hospitals but also to home-visit nursing care for which a protocol has been developed, and the results have been verified as this theory being effective through studies. Furthermore, the protocol developed for home-visit nursing care has been successfully incorporated into an electronic recording system, which is now in operation throughout the nation. In the academic domain, researchers have reported on the development of new educational programs based on this theory. As an example of the extent of international acceptance beyond Japan, a textbook based on this theory has been translated into Taiwanese, and its use is becoming widely accepted in Taiwan.

Performing Diagnosis and Assessment

Setting a goal is definitely required for assessment. A physician is responsible for determining treatment policies for patients by using an assessment process. Consider a "diagnosis" made in clinical arenas. On what does a physician base a diagnosis? For example, the physician needs to find out whether a patient has pneumonia and, if so, whether it is infectious or noninfectious and if it is bacterial or viral pneumonia. If it is bacterial pneumonia, the physician also must identify the bacteria responsible to ensure appropriate drug selection. However, when determining care policies for patients with pneumonia to ease breathing, the physician does not need to identify the bacteria, strictly. It is clear that the physician must separate patients with pulmonary tuberculosis from others in order to maintain a secure medical environment.

A sound basic policy reflecting both clinical inference and assessment is *to determine the condition of a patient*. In the case of aftereffects from cerebral infarction, for example, patients are all given the same disease name, but the conditions of daily life for each patient can vary. Of course, knowing a patient's history of cerebral infarction greatly helps the physician predict the patient's future status.

Physicians are required to assess a patient's condition to provide the proper care to provide. Efforts invested do not need to go beyond what is required. Patients and medical staff should avoid unnecessary waste of energy, which is necessary for the effective operation of clinical practice. The important point is to improve the quality and effectiveness of the staff's work.

Monitoring-Intervention-Monitoring

Sometimes *intervention* involves *not* taking action. Nursing intervention is defined as a series of activities that nurses must take in specific circumstances. However, not taking action also can be considered an intervention. Staying away from patients is not a visible activity and is hardly recognized as an interventional activity. In fact, monitoring is not a visible activity either, but it should be conducted before and after every care activity. Thus, the set of monitoring-intervention-monitoring activities cannot be separated.

In fact, this set of monitoring-intervention-monitoring activities is conducted unconsciously. Although nurses have a nursing plan, they do not force patients to follow the plan when their conditions or feelings change. Nurses must always monitor patients after interventional activities. As a matter of course in nursing, *not doing anything* is not the same as *unconsciously doing things*, and *doing things* is not the same as *unconsciously doing things*. Doing something is not what is required. Nurses must determine what to do and when as well as what not to do. Not only doing things but also not doing anything is a part of nursing intervention. The important point is to be fully aware of this principle.

LAYERED MODEL OF LIFE FUNCTION

The ultimate goal for nursing care is to find a way to provide livelihood support for patients. Nurses need to observe how people live, who they are, and what aspect of their environment or situation affects their daily lives. Nursing requires keen observation of various factors and a global perspective. The necessity of physical assessment in professional nursing is closely associated with the essential role of nursing practice: to provide support to patients.

There are various methods of providing livelihood support to patients. For example, social workers are responsible for helping individuals find a way to interact with society through social support. To provide patients with livelihood support, physicians employ invasive treatment and medical therapy. Physical therapists use a rehabilitative approach for improved physical and mental functions, and nutritionists give patients nutritional advice for a good balance of mind and body. Nurses discuss and coordinate these actions to provide appropriate nursing environments to assist patients' recovery.

How to Monitor Patients' Daily Lives

Because livelihood support for patients is a central and essential role for nursing practice, visible nursing activities should be related to patients' daily life support. To fulfill this role, nurses are required to monitor patients in various daily situations, for example, whether they are able to eat adequately and keep themselves clean. Monitoring that is interpreted from the viewpoint of the activities of daily living (ADL) makes it is easy to recognize what monitoring indicates.

People cannot live without associating with others and their surrounding environment. How people communicate with others and adapt to the surrounding environment is fundamental to life. Nurses are expected to intervene in this area when necessary. Nurses who monitor patients from an environmental point of view recognize that monitoring activities always overlap.

There are two types of human system functioning: one is a person's conscious use of the body to try to do something; the other is a person's unconscious use of the body to avoid a risk. Sometimes, the latter one automatically works regardless of the person's intention because the intention could bring danger to the body.

If the human system function, which works regardless of the person's intention, is disabled, that person faces mortal danger. Vital life functions work regardless of a person's will. These functions constitute the backbone of the entire body and are connected with every aspect of daily life. When trying to rest, exercise, or eat, a person can never stop breathing or bowel peristalsis. Even while sleeping, nutrient absorption cannot be stopped. Any attempt to stop bowel peristalsis will most certainly be in vain.

The basic premise common to various aspects of daily life is that the human body survives as an organism. From the viewpoint of supporting the individual's livelihood, vital life functions always interact with every event of daily life. In other words, monitoring to sustain life is repeatedly conducted at every single event of daily life.

SUMMARY

The theoretical framework was developed from the author's background both in medicine and physiology, with specific applications to nursing knowledge development from the perspective of the need for assessment of life functioning. A hierarchy of factors within this life function theory is identified. There is a need for further development of the theoretical perspective both empirically and applied to clinical nursing practice.

REFERENCES

Mitoma, R. (2009). *Development of a learning support program for home visiting nurses to utilize physical assessment skills on respiratory system.* Doctoral Dissertation, St. Luke's College of Nursing, Japan.

OECD. (2015), *Nurses* (indicator). doi: 10.1787/283e64de-en (Accessed on 09 February 2015).

Tsai, Y. (2013). *Physical assessment guidebook.* Ho-Chi Book Publishing Co., Taipei, Taiwan.

Yamauchi, T. (2004). *Physical assessment,* DVD Vol. 1–10, Video Pack Nippon, Tokyo, Japan.

Yamauchi, T. (2005). *Physical assessment guidebook.* Igaku-Shoin Publishing, Tokyo, Japan.

Yamauchi, T. (2011). *Physical assessment guidebook,* 2nd ed. Igaku-Shoin Publising, Tokyo, Japan.

Yamauchi, T. (2011). *Vital signs,* DVD Vol. 1–3, Video Pack Nippon, Tokyo, Japan.

Yamauchi, T. (2012). *Sign and symptom,* DVD Vol. 1–8, Video Pack Nippon, Tokyo, Japan.

Yamauchi, T. (2014). *Physical assessment workbook.* Igaku-Shoin Publishing, Tokyo, Japan.

Yamauchi, T., & Okamoto, S. (2009). *Home visiting nursing; Assessment protocol.* Chuo-Hohki Publishing, Tokyo, Japan.

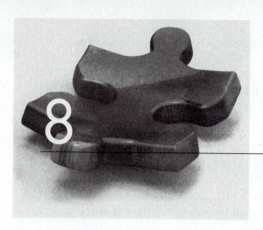

Spain: Barcelona's Clinic Hospital Nursing Model

Roser Cadena, Emili Comas, Teresa Fusté, Pedro Sanz, Montserrat Valverde, and Adelaida Zabalegui on behalf of the technical committee Nursing Direction of Hospital Clinic Barcelona

INTRODUCTION

Longer life expectancy and advances in science and technology have affected the nature and prevalence of illnesses and conditions, increasing the complexity of patient care. This population shift requires making changes in nursing practice methods that reflect evidence-based care and best practice. According to data from the Catalan Autonomous Government (Generalitat of Catalonia), 32% of the population covered by the Barcelona Clinic Hospital (BCH) is more than 65 years old of whom 60% are men and 40% are women (Gencat, 2012). Life expectancy in Catalonia is higher than in other Spanish and European regions. The average age for men is 76.3 years, and for women is 83.4 years (Idescat, 2012). These social and demographic changes in addition to the increased efficiency of clinical resources have challenged the health care system's ability to provide efficient and effective continuing care. Changes in the way health is managed for individuals and their significant others have been embraced by BCH and have led to changes in nursing practice, new management settings, and essential restructuring of the organization. Currently, nursing professionals require continuous development and comprehensive expertise in order to reach excellence in their practice and meet their patients' complex needs.

BCH was founded in 1906; it has the dual role of serving the community and acting as a tertiary care facility. It is the main supplier of public health in its area within Barcelona city and provides service to a population of 540,725 inhabitants (32% of Barcelona's total population). In addition, BCH, a high-complexity tertiary care hospital with an annual budget of €500 million, provides high technological medical services such as liver transplants to 7,200,000 inhabitants. The hospital has 770 beds and 4,500 staff members of whom 55% belong to the department of nursing with 1,301 (28.9% of the total hospital workforce) permanent nursing employees.

BCH provides many important services for patients, not only in Catalonia but also throughout Spain and other countries. It offers all types of health care treatments with the exception of pediatric care and burn management. In 2012, the hospital had 41,826 discharges (including outpatient surgery) with a complexity index of 2.18%, 109,330 emergency admissions, 23,656 surgical procedures, 376 transplants, 590 knee replacements, 3,316 newborn deliveries, 108,167 initial assessments, and 99,567 hospital follow-ups.

To continue to provide the comprehensive care and treatment, BCH participated in the management of primary care centers, developed mental health services in the community, and established alliances with other centers to provide continuing care and meet social and long-term health needs in the community.

As a teaching hospital, BCH is a role model at national and international levels and maintains excellence in clinical education, training, and research. It offers continuous annual teaching and learning activities and accommodates 319 junior nurses and doctors in a specialization teaching period called *residency*, 258 trainee doctors from other institutions, 284 professionals in work experience, 103 accredited courses, and 30 residency graduation awards. In 2013, the number of nursing students performing their clinical training at BCH was 953. Of these, 532 students belonged to the bachelor of sciences nursing program, and each student practiced in the hospital during a period of two to three months. In addition, 187 nursing students attended postgraduate courses, including master's degree programs; the remaining nursing students were enrolled in other undergraduate programs such as nutrition and physiotherapy.

Regarding research activities, in 2013, the hospital produced 1,005 original publications with a total impact factor of 5.595 points and an average of 5.56 points in the impact factor index. The impact factor is a measure reflecting the average number of citations to recent articles published in that journal and it is frequently used as a proxy for the relative importance of a journal within its field. The BCH also had 578 active research projects and 58 visiting professors from other institutions doing clinical research.

BCH has always been a ground-breaking center. In 1995, it devised the Prisma Project, a unique organizational model (Font, Piqué, Guerra & Rodés, 2008). This model was implemented as a new structure for the hospital by clustering each department with other medical services that had the same clinical expertise; these new organizations were called *institutes*. They had a common purpose to provide patient-focused care that is more personalized and specialized for its users. This new arrangement enforced a less centralized management and allowed nurses and physicians to have increased responsibility and more independent management of resources. The Prisma Project entailed a completely new design for the hospital's health care processes and put patients at the center of the care. Its objective was to improve the quality of care while decreasing hospital cost. This innovative reform had three main principles:

- To group patients according to their requirements and specific characteristics
- To organize services to meet the needs of patients and professionals
- To decentralize the organization whenever possible

For the past 10 years, BCH has received the award for the best of the Top 20 Hospitals in Spain, a prize given to leading Spanish hospitals that assess management and quality in different areas such as direct management, women's health, and respiratory medicine among others. BCH has an ongoing commitment and effort to improve services and hospital processes. Delivery of patient processes is constantly evaluated and improved in light of their efficiency, effectiveness, and flexibility. Today, one of BCH's main goals is to increase its efficiency by redesigning its structure and health care management. The development of a new nursing model was required to provide guidance at each stage of the care planning process in line with the evolving hospital's philosophy.

A new nursing model, the BCH nursing model, was included in BCH's 2010 strategic plan. The model had a progressive implementation method in the hospital and was flexible to make suitable adjustments according to the characteristic of each hospital institute and center.

BARCELONA'S CLINIC HOSPITAL (BCH) NURSING MODEL

In 1994, BCH's nursing department agreed to implement Virginia Henderson's (VH) nursing model of needs as the framework for the University of Barcelona Nursing School. In Spain, the VH model is the most used nursing model in hospitals; 82% of nursing schools have adopted it in their core curriculums (Santos, 2013). However, the implementation of the VH model did not fulfill expectations and was barely implemented at BCH. Only patient assessments were based on the VH model.

In 2011, BCH participated with 16 other countries in the international research study RN4CAST-Nurse forecasting in Europe (RN4CAST, 2013). This study was conducted by Linda Aiken's research team from the U.S. Center for Health Outcomes and Policy Research at the University of Pennsylvania and was led in Europe by Walter Sermeus from the Centre for Health Services and Nursing Research, KU Leuven in Belgium. The purpose of this research study was to gain deeper knowledge and understanding of how nursing staff perceive their work environment. Nurses were asked about the quality of care that they provided to service users. The results of this research study showed that nurses working at BCH felt the need to be guided by an appropriate nursing model of care. They required a comprehensive and meaningful vision of how they should provide nursing care. As a result of this study, BCH's nursing department saw an exceptional opportunity to implement a new model of care to improve the care given to the hospital's patients.

Accordingly, the nursing department began to develop the new BCH nursing model of care whose objectives were accepted to:

- Improve health care quality and safety
- Encourage a strong learning environment that supports expert knowledge and innovation
- Prioritize professional nursing development
- Enhance evidence-based practice
- Promote nursing leadership within the hospital

The new nursing model provides a framework for future practice. The 2010 BCH strategic nursing plan identified the mission, vision, and values of the nursing department as well as feasible and desirable targets, strategic planning, and quality improvements. The following nursing model elements were set to guide the organization's strategic planning and performance assessment activities. The mission, vision, and values are the foundational concepts that assure the nurses daily work guidance.

Mission

One guideline was to guarantee the patients high-quality care while maintaining safety, respecting patients' privacy, respecting and protecting their rights and dignity, and enabling them to recover and adjust to their new health status. Nurses must provide aid to all vulnerable people by engaging in health promotion and disease prevention and giving maximum comfort to patients from admission to end of life. Also, they provide counseling and allow a patient's family, caregivers, and significant others to be involved in the care process.

Vision

Nursing staff endeavor to become an international role model for the health care field within the framework of BCH as a highly complex tertiary care and community hospital.

Values

Humanitarianism (respect, participation, and trust), interdisciplinary collaboration, scientific rigor, and excellence in patient care are the stated values.

METHODOLOGY FOR THE DEVELOPMENT OF THE BCH NURSING MODE

Phase 1

In February 2011, the nursing team held monthly meetings to address three main questions: What do patients need? How do we deliver care? And how would we like to deliver care?

A literature review was performed to give the nursing team up-to-date knowledge of others' relevant work. The review identified a gap in the nursing care provided at BCH, and the nursing team acknowledged that the VH model of care developed in the 1950s was not effective for the BCH context and did not respond to patient's needs. Thus, the nurses' level of engagement was affected and appropriate responses to patient's demands and expectations were compromised.

The nursing department proposed that the new BCH nursing model have a few simple rules to implement at several different patient units with small changes that could have a significant impact on improving care and patients' experiences.

To gather the necessary information to create the BCH nursing model, a complex intervention method was used; it included a total of approximately 250 participants (nurses, patients, physicians, and health care assistants). The mixed method approach included:

- *Focus groups*: A leading external expert conducted three focus groups attended by 22 nurses, 10 nursing unit managers, and two health care assistants who participated in analyzing the care that nurses were then providing and the care that they would like to provide.

- *In-depth interviews and non-participative observation*: This involved a total of 22 one-to-one interviews of nurses and physicians (morning and afternoon shifts) at 11 different units (five medical units, five surgical units, and one mixed unit) to explore the expert's opinion and to triangulate this knowledge through observation.
- *Patient feedback questionnaires*: These questionnaires gathered the views of 90 inpatients before their discharge regarding the care they received during their hospitalization.
- *Retrospective analysis of patients' complaints*: From all data collected between 2010 and 2011, complaints from 234 patients were analyzed retrospectively.

Following the analysis of the data, the nursing department could identify six key points to incorporate into the principles of the BCH nursing model. The principles established were as follows: patient empowerment, use of evidence-based practices and best practices, effective communication with the multidisciplinary team, improvement of professional nurses' competence, implementation of advanced nursing practice roles, and encouragement of nursing leadership.

These six key principles were presented to all the chief nurses of each BCH institute and center and to care managers in May 2012. A workshop with 120 participants was held to analyze and discuss these principles and to determine nursing managers' agreement of them. Furthermore, the nursing department agreed to appoint 12 additional working groups to learn about and further analyze the implementation of these principles in different hospital units.

Phase 2

With the previous objectives in mind, the implementation of the BCH nursing model evolved to a second phase in which 12 working groups from two different areas were formed. One area was in charge of analyzing the nursing model's implementation by clinical units such as intensive care or emergency unit, and the second area considered the model's implementation in common instrumental components, for example, communication, supervision, organization of care, quality, and safety.

- Six teams worked on the practical implementation of the model in complex medical and surgical services with different team dynamics such as operating rooms, intensive care units, emergency units, diagnostic imaging centers, laboratory units, day care units, integrated care units, and home hospitalization units.

- An additional six working groups studied the practical implementation of the BCH nursing model in different instrumental components of care to provide practical means to accomplish the best possible patient care. These components were explored in different units to challenge the difficulties in the practical application of the six key elements of the nursing model. The components were organization of patient care, communication between nurse and health care assistant and between nurse and physician, general supervision, care quality, and safety. Possibilities of enhancing advanced nursing roles and communication and information technology tools were also explored.

The results of phase 2 were presented at the 6th Annual BCH Nursing Conference in October 2013 and were supported by medical directors of all BCH institutes and centers. In addition, this model received the award for the best organizational innovation at the MIHealth 2014 in Barcelona.

PRINCIPLES OF BCH NURSING CARE

Patient Empowerment

The patient empowerment approach is well suited to expand patient-centered care and patient participation in making informed decisions and in taking an active role in their health decisions. Patient health education and information has become an important part of therapy and patient empowerment. In addition, health promotion allows patients and caregivers to become active participants in their health care and enable patients to make their own treatment choices. One of the nurses' responsibilities is to develop educational interventions oriented to enhance patients' knowledge of and to support the active involvement of patients and their families in the design of care plans and decision-making options for treatment.

The concept of empowerment first appeared in the 1970s in the field of social and psychological education. Rappaport (1981, 1988) defined a new model for the social psychology of empowerment, and Gibson (1991) subsequently applied this concept to the health care environment. Gibson believed that patient empowerment can be achieved through education that allows patients to make decisions that could improve their biopsychosocial well-being. A problem-solving attitude adjustment raises patients' consciousness regarding their own health and eases the management of their health related issues (Rankinnen et al., 2007).

BCH defines the concept of patient education and information as the process of enabling adults to make their own decisions based on information about their own health and act accordingly. The empowered patient is an educated patient who uses that knowledge to make preferred health choices.

Recent studies have defined six dimensions of empowerment that influence daily activities as physiological, functional, social, experiential, ethical, and financial (Leino-Kilpi et al., 2005). The physiological dimension of empowerment is based on a patient's ability to recognize the signs and symptoms of the condition, allowing him or her to take control of his or her own health. The functional dimension allows patients to control their situation with regard to their own mobility. The social dimension empowers patients to maintain a social role despite their disease. The experiential aspect enables patients to draw on their previous experiences to take charge of their problem. The ethical dimension is experienced as unique and makes patients feel that they are receiving appropriate attention that guarantees their well-being. The final dimension is the financial one, which considers an individual's economic funding to fulfill his or her health requirements. This approach is included in the BCH nursing model.

Placing patients' needs first at the core of care and empowering them through education and information is a new view implemented by the BCH nursing model. By integrating this new approach in clinical practice, BCH enables patients to participate in the decision-making process regarding their own health with the guidance of health care professionals. To maximize self-care and self-management, the BCH nursing model promotes appropriate patient education and structured training for patients and caregivers.

EVIDENCE-BASED AND BEST PRACTICES

Evidence-based nursing care is an approach to making quality decisions and providing nursing care based on personal clinical expertise in combination with the most current, relevant research available on the topic. According to Sackett (1996), this approach is the conscientious, explicit, and judicious use of current best evidence to make decisions about the care of individual patients. It is based on four general concepts: research, clinical experience, users' preferences/values, and available resources. This approach enables patients and nurses to make informed decisions about health care and promote a better quality of care. Also, it enables health care providers to understand the comparative effectiveness of different types of care to ensure the best use of resources. To maintain and improve the level of professional competence, nurses' daily work requires the use of critical thinking and reflective practice.

This new vision of nursing practice provides the best expert evidence obtained from relevant clinical research and makes nurses rethink current educational programs. The evidence-based clinical practice has influenced BCH nursing knowledge, organization, and clinical practice in general.

Maintain Effective Communication with the Team Members

Communication is a key element for teamwork. Effective communication allows team members to understand what roles they play. Poor team communication could waste health care professionals' time and efforts as the result of undertaking unnecessary tasks, duplicating work, and not understanding duties and responsibilities. The miscommunications, or lack of communication, could lead to conflicts and damage the trust relationship among the professionals. People who fail to communicate effectively can ultimately not have the necessary facts to perform their duties properly.

Good communication combined with strong organizational support, qualified leadership, and comprehensive objectives could lead to successful teamwork. Outstanding team communication can assist continuity of care by building a safe environment and increasing quality of care.

Improve Nurses' Professional Competence

Nurses deliver and provide services independently and within the multidisciplinary team. As team members, they provide support during all of the aspects of care and contribute their knowledge and overall view of a patient's condition. Also, nurses coordinate the care between the patient and other health, social, primary, and secondary care professionals. In addition, nurses are essential participants in providing all aspects of patients' care.

Nurses' professional interest goes beyond health issues. Their vision is to provide holistic care for patients and their families and significant others. Nurses are involved from referral to discharge for the duration of patients' admission to the hospital. Nurses are the most suitable professionals to keep track of and monitor patients' progress. Also, they are highly qualified professionals who coordinate complex processes that occur throughout disease management when intervention of different professionals is required.

Nurses are responsible for patients' well-being and establishing an effective coordination of care within BCH. They are able to improve the quality of care given to patients by improving their knowledge, skills, and attitudes.

Education grants have enabled BCH to facilitate advanced nursing practice and enable nurses to improve their competencies. Also, the hospital has implemented a professional development plan (PDP) that integrates five levels of nursing. The plan evaluates nurses' performance in different areas such as knowledge, skills, experience, and educational research. This encourages nurses to build specific competencies and participate in continuous training and development. The PDP recognizes the excellence in nursing practice and allows BCH nurses to achieve desirable professional promotions. For instance, to reach the highest level (nurse expert), a nurse must have completed her or his Ph.D. and a research project as a principal investigator. The PDP is an encouraging element for the nursing professional development and a motivation towards excellence of practice.

Implement Advanced Nursing Practice Roles and Encourage Nursing Leadership

BCH nursing leadership has been approached from different views:

- *Nurse managers' leadership*: When nurse managers use empowerment strategies, they create safer environments for other professionals and promote efficiency and effectiveness in the area of care. The International Council of Nurses acknowledges that reforms of the health care systems are taking place around the world and that nurse managers must have the opportunity to lead this change (MacPhee, Skelton-Green, Bouthillette, & Suryaprakash, 2011).
- *Staff nurse leadership*: Nurses must focus on supporting the patient, managing and coordinating care, maintaining the patient's safety and dignity, promoting health, and acting as the patient's reference.
- *Advanced practice nursing leadership*: This enables nurses to lead in specific areas of expertise such as anesthesia or mental health at BCH. In Spain, this advanced nursing role lacks a legal framework for practice. At BCH, the nursing department is innovative in implementing some of these roles.

Nurses should consider different leadership approaches regarding patients' care and collaborate with other allied health professionals. BCH has very competent nurses who are able to deal with professional challenges and act as real leaders and to influence the social, economic, and political aspects affecting the health care they provide. They seek to improve health care in the society and cost effectively increase the quality of life for individuals.

BCH NURSING MODEL'S KEY ELEMENTS

The Person

A *person* is considered a biological, psychological, social, cultural, and spiritual being involved in a dynamic environment in which he or she constantly interacts and plans to improve both his or her health and quality of life. Nurses are closely linked to the person's family and surrounding cultural, political, and social values. People have rights and duties. Their rights must be respected, but they must collaborate in the health process according to their skills and knowledge and have a commitment to keep a healthy environment (CatSalut, 1997).

Health

Health is a dynamic and continuous state of balance and adaptation that depends on a person's perception and therefore could have different meanings. It is a process that lasts the entire lifetime (CatSalut, 1997).

The Environment

The *environment* is the framework in which the person, family, and community coexist. It has several dimensions including social, economic, political, cultural, and spiritual. It can represent a source of support for development but also entails a potential risk (CatSalut, 1997).

The Role of Caring in the Nursing Profession

Nursing care contributes in specific ways to the health promotion, well-being, and quality of life of the person, the family, and the environment. Nursing activities focus on the person's specific needs whenever he or she has a health problem. The nursing profession offers care for the person in all dimensions within a framework of interdisciplinary collaboration.

Optimal nursing care is based on humanistic values and scientific knowledge. It allows the patient and caregivers to take responsibility for their own health. Appropriate nursing care includes the knowledge and skills to maintain and/or improve a patient's health and to encourage education and self-care.

RELATION BETWEEN THE MODEL'S PRINCIPLES AND ITS MAIN COMPONENTS

Research

The Nursing Research Council's strategic plan is to promote nursing research to improve evidence-based practice. The objectives of BCH's nursing department are to encourage nurses who are interested in research, increase the number of publications and research projects, create alliances inside and outside BCH, support professionals who are at the top of their field, and address new areas of research. Efforts have been made to support research by encouraging nurses to seek advanced degrees.

The BCH nursing department is currently participating in a European project led by H. Leino-Kilpi from Turku University of Finland. The project's main goal is to increase patient empowerment and develop assessment tools in order to learn about educational interventions through two experiences. By empowering patients who suffer from osteoarthritis, the first project aims to encourage patients and families to participate in improving their biophysiological, functional, and social well-being. Patients and their families take part in creating solutions to their problems and gain specific skills that enable them to handle their health issues. The project seeks to improve patients' satisfaction while cutting hospital costs. The second project is to implement the empowerment of oncology patients by developing a tool for health care professionals to assist oncology patients in making informed decisions.

Education

An education unit in BCH has been created with the assistance of Barcelona University Nursing School. The two organizations have worked together with a common approach to nursing education and practice. This collaboration on the bachelor of science degree in nursing integrates professors of nursing and clinical expertise. This joint effort is a four-year scientific program within the medical school of Barcelona University (Zabalegui et al., 2006; Zabalegui & Cabrera, 2010). In addition, the two organizations have created an advanced nursing practice program with hospital funding through grants-in-aid for postgraduate education.

BCH also collaborates with the Nursing Science Department at Turku University (Finland). This collaboration was created to allow the nursing department at both the BCH and the Turku University to better understand different nursing systems from the perspective of nursing clinical specialists, managers, and leaders to improve evidence-based practice. BCH nursing staff regularly attend an advanced training course on patients' empowerment under Helena Leino-Kilpi's supervision in Finland. In addition, staff nurses from Turku University's specialized center come to BCH to gain work experience and further their practical education.

Professional Practice

Regarding clinical practice, the guideline for nursing care organization in units seeks to implement the BCH nursing model's values in a comprehensive way by using health teams as a key component. A team of nurses from each BCH institute created a guideline which had the purpose of assessing and auditing compliance with clinical governance and hospital policies.

In addition, nurses' delegates contribute to all hospital committees as "full partners" at every level of hierarchy. The BCH nursing model acknowledges nurses' autonomy and introduces integrated care units, which are educational units for chronic patients, such as those suffering with diabetes or Chronic Obstructive Pulmonary Disease (COPD). The model also promotes advanced practice roles for nurses characterized by their autonomy in decision making based on specific training and clinical expertise.

BCH also has created a nursing research committee to emphasize strong professional commitment to evidence-based practice. The committee integrates nurses from each institute and department by having them participate in all the hospital's committee sessions as well as decision and management departments to ensure that the nurses' point of view regarding the management of processes in the hospital is being heard.

In addition, a program for the evaluation of nursing competencies at high levels has been developed to empower nurses and their teams. The annual assessment of the nursing competencies considers six different areas: planning and organization, team management, resource management, communication, nursing quality of care, and hospital commitment. This evaluation system allows nursing management leaders and their teams to expand. Other goals of the assessment are to create an educational evolution and to identify areas of leadership improvement. Under the new BCH nursing model, nursing professionals are allowed more responsibility and autonomy. Moreover, every four years, BCH evaluates lead nurses' performance to decide whether they are able to continue in their management positions.

Considering the importance of assessment, BCH nursing management, with other institutions from the Catalonian Hospitals Coalition, is leading in assessing nursing care quality. Being a part of this association allows nurses to compare care and evaluate standards of practice.

REFERENCES

CatSalut (1997). *La professió d'infermeria. Principis i línies estratègiques*. Consell Assessor d'Infermeria Generalitat de Catalunya.

Font, D., Piqué, J. M., Guerra, F., & Rodés, J. (2008). Implantación de la gestión clínica en la organización hospitalaria. *Medicina Clínica, 130*(9), 351–356.

Generalitat de Catalunya (2012). *Memoria 201*. CatSalut. Servei Catalá de la Salut. Departament de Salut. http://www20.gencat.cat/docs/salut/Minisite/catsalut/publicacions/docs/memoria_catsalut2012_castellano.pdf

Gibson, C. H. (1991). A concept analysis of empowerment. *Journal of Advanced Nursing*, *16*, 354–361.

Indescat. (2012). Estructura de la población. Anuari estadístic de la población. http://www .idescat.cat/pub/?id=aec&n=27

Leino-Kilpi, H., Johansson, K., Heikkiene, K., Kaljonen, A., Virtanen, H., & Salanterä, S. (2005). Patient education and health-related quality of life: Surgical hospital patients as a case in point. *Journal of Nursing Care Quality*, *20*(4), 307–316.

MacPhee, M., Skelton-Green, J., Bouthillette, F., & Suryaprakash, N. (2011). An empowerment framework for nursing leadership development: Supporting evidence. *Journal of Advanced Nursing*, *10*, 159–169.

Rankinnen, S., Salantera, S., Heikkinen, K., Johansson, K., Kaljonen, A., Virtanen, H., & Leino-Kilpi, H. (2007). Ambulatory orthopaedic surgery patients' knowledge expectations and perceptions of received knowledge. *Journal of Advanced Nursing*, *60*, 270–278.

Rappaport, J. (1981). In praise of paradox: A social policy of empowerment over prevention. *American Journal of Community Psychology*, *9*(1), 1–25.

Rappaport, J. (1988). Terms of empowerment/exemplars of prevention: Toward a theory for community psychology. *American Journal of Community Psychology*, *15*(2), 121–148.

RN4CAST Consorcium. (2013). Prevalence, patterns and predictors of nursing care left undone in European hospitals: Results from the multi country cross-sectional RN4CAST study. *BMJ Quality & Safety Online First*. doi:10.1136/bmjqs.2013-002318

Sackett, D. L. (1996). Medicina basada en la evidencia: Lo que es y no. *British Medical Journal*, 312, 71–72.

Santos, S. (2013). *Factores determinantes del uso de los modelos teóricos en la práctica enfermera*. Tesis Doctoral. Jaume I University (Valencia – Spain)

Zabalegui, A., & Cabrera, E. (2010). Economic crisis and nursing in Spain. *Journal of Nursing Management, 18*, 505–508.

Zabalegui, A., Macia, L., Marquez, J., Ricomá, R., Nuin, C., Mariscal, I., Moncho, J. (2006). Changes in nursing education in the European Union. *Journal of Nursing Scholarship*, *38*(2), 114–118.

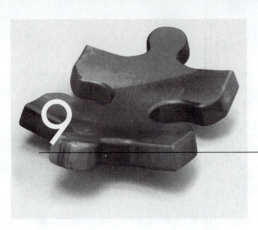

South Korea: Theory of Interpersonal Caring

Susie Kim, Haeok Lee, and Younhee Kang

INTRODUCTION: BASIC ELEMENTS OF INTERPERSONAL CARING THEORY

The theory of interpersonal caring (IC) was originally based on Peplau's *personal relations theory*, which involves both caring and interpersonal relationships, and was built inductively from the patients' experiences of "being cared for" (Peplau, 1952, 1992). The IC theory developed is a patient-centered, patient-focused, and patient-oriented form of caring. This IC theory extended Peplau's theory of the nurse–patient relationship from *doing to* to *doing with* patients by providing the context for what this means and how it is done.

IC theory is deeply rooted in the notion of mental illness in South Korea in the 1980s and 1990s (Kim, 1989; Kim & Ae, 1999; Kim & Berry, 1997). South Korea had no mental health act until 1995, and many mentally ill people commonly stayed for long terms in institutions, such as sanatoriums, and secluded healing places. Mental illness in Korean culture is stigmatized and is generally looked down upon; those who suffer it are seen as being at the bottom of society. Hence, Koreans are highly reluctant to talk openly about mental health problems for fear of being socially stigmatized and discriminated against. The IC theory was achieved within this sociocultural context in which the developer lived with, taught, and studied with mentally handicapped individuals. The IC theory was developed from the identification of their life experiences (Kim, 1989; Kim, 1997; Kim, 2000; Kim 2002; Kim, 2012). It specifically addresses the lives of mentally handicapped individuals in their life settings and consequently provides a different perspective of the mentally handicapped in the hope of improving nursing practice for them. The IC theory helps nurses and other caring professionals to learn that the ultimate goal of caring is to help patients to realize the source of their inner strengths as well as their sense of self-worth and self-esteem. This realization leads them to find meaning and direction for their existence.

KEY CONCEPTS OF KIM'S INTERPERSONAL CARING THEORY

Definition and Discretion of Nursing

This theory defines *caring* as the primary aspect of nursing. It is the core and essence of the theory. Caring in nursing is a way to empower the sick and the needy.

Interpersonal Caring as a Basic Concept

Interpersonal caring involves both caring and developing a person-to-person relationship that is the essence of nursing. It involves compassion-based therapeutic actions/behaviors developed through the collaborative partnership process developed between nurse (care provider) and patient (care receiver). It enables the patient to achieve a sense of self-worth and self-esteem, which motivates him or her to comply with various treatment regimens for optimal well-being and wholeness. The concept sees caring not only as acknowledging wellness and wholeness, but also applying it and passing it to patients with genuine love and concern. Interpersonal caring emerges through trust based on compassion, a deepening and qualitative transformation of the relationship between nurse and patient, and direct and indirect interactions between the two. IC can be witnessed in the collaborative nurse–patient relationship that is based on mutual connection, trust, and respect for one's right to be himself or herself. In particular, in the context of psychiatric nursing situations, IC as a therapeutic process facilitates the patient's sense of self-worth and self-esteem, which provides the inner strength to move the patient toward wholeness, integrity, and connectedness. The nurse in the relationship does not exercise power over or dominate the patient but collaborates and helps.

The Ten Key Components Identified by the Kim Theory of Interpersonal Care

The key elements of the theory follow.

1. *Noticing* is the act of comprehensively recognizing someone's existence by taking an interest in that person. It requires the skill of a nurse to use his or her mental abilities and attitudes through sensory information gained from sight, hearing, smell, taste, and touch in order to become aware of the subtle changes, expressions, appearances, feelings, desires, and needs of a patient or family. By noticing these, the nurse comes to know a patient, which involves simultaneously recognizing the realms of the physical, mental, social, spiritual, and aesthetic.

2. *Participating* means that a nurse joins in and does an activity with a patient that is needed to maintain and promote her or his health. It requires the skill of simultaneously observing the other person's physical, psychological, and spiritual dimensions and being involved in their experience. Participatory actions help patients to recognize how supportive someone can be in the distressing realities they face and eventually can help them to deal with, and overcome, their problems.

3. *Sharing* is the act of unconditional readiness that leads to an openness of one's innermost self. It involves mutual disclosure of life's most valued dimensions, such as feelings, thoughts, experiences, knowledge (information), plans, and concerns—in short, every good and bad thing we think about ourselves—and an open discussion of them. The nature of sharing is found in an old Korean saying, "When sorrow is shared, it halves, and when joy is shared it doubles." Through sharing, some patients experience the "rediscovery of trust" as a therapeutic turning point.

4. *Active listening* means consciously and intently paying attention to what truly needs to be heard. It is the act of listening to another person's words with all of one's heart and genuineness of attitude. It entails hearing not only the spoken words but also the speaker's inner thoughts and feelings; it seeks to discover the meaning behind actions and words. It is the act of paying close attention to understand each word and its meaning.

5. *Companioning* means joining in the solitary path a person is taking. It is attending to the other's experience and holding each other. Companioning is extending oneself to the other person by "being present with," and caring is communicated through companioning or the presence of the caring person in a nursing situation.

It is the nurse encountering the patient as a unique person within the context of the nursing situation. This is accomplished through words, actions, feelings, and closeness to make the patient feel emotionally supported.

6. *Complimenting* involves acknowledging the other person's strengths and potential and expressing gratitude for them. It includes encouraging, trusting, affirming, boosting self-confidence, promoting growth and development, and supporting the person's strengths. Complimenting supports patients and inspires them to have courage and a can-do spirit in their daily lives, work, and relationships with other patients, family members, and health care providers.

7. *Comforting* exhibits an empathetic attitude toward the patient. It is the action of understanding and comforting the person in his or her sadness or pain. It involves the skill of acknowledging the person's feelings from his or her perspective, of accepting the person, of becoming an unconditional ally, and of pulling together his or her greater strength instead of defending a third party who caused hurt. Comforting is a skill of providing what a patient needs, offering additional strengths and a shelter.

8. *Hoping* is the act of infusing energy or sources of strength in another person. Hope is "a mental state characterized by the desire to gain an end or accomplish a goal combined with some degree of expectation that what is desired or sought is attainable" (Travelbee, 1971), and it is related to dependence on others, choice, wishes, trust, perseverance, and courage. Hoping entails offering love to the person in the midst of her or his despair or disappointments. It connects with a loved one and can include connecting the patient to nature.

9. *Forgiving* is the act of acknowledging wrong conduct and seeking leniency with a genuine expression of saying "I am sorry, and please forgive me." In expressing remorse and seeking forgiveness, there should be no attempt to explain or make excuses. It is pure grace when that forgiveness is taken. It comes out of love; it touches lives. There is no easy method; it is simply a matter of the heart. Forgiveness can transform people into global communities.

10. *Accepting* is the act of acknowledging and receiving the patient as she or he is without any judgment or criticism. It contains the actions of listening, understanding, allowing, and concurring with the person as if in her or his shoes. Accepting needs willing involvement with a patient with a constant and mutual

unfolding of the nurse–patient relationship. The strength of courage needed by the person in the nursing situation to practice acceptance can be awe inspiring.

Definition and Description of Person(s)

In the IC theory, *persons* are dynamic human beings with bio-psycho/ emotional-social-spiritual needs. It defines human beings as growing, living, and capable of self-actualization through interpersonal caring.

Definition and Description of Environment

The IC theory's concept of the *environment* is assumed to be the internal and external resources and the surrounding energy field that influences the patient's quality of living. The nursing situation is the environment in the theory and is interpreted as a shared living experience, a relationship built upon "caring" between nurse and patient. When this happens, IC occurs.

Definition and Description of Health

Health, in the IC theory, is a state full of positive energy that includes knowledge, strength, will, and love for abundant life. It also expands the definition of health to include both the physically handicapped and the mentally handicapped.

Analysis and Evaluation

Interpersonal caring is the outcome of it's developer's reflections, studies, and practice with patients, families, students, and colleagues over many years. It describes, explains, and predicts that human caring can be effectively demonstrated and practiced interpersonally. It enhances the well-being and wholeness of human beings.

RELATIONSHIP AMONG THE MODEL'S CONCEPTS AND COMPONENTS

As discussed, the IC model contains 10 interpersonal caring techniques (ICTs) to help mentally ill patients rediscover motivation and a zest for life as well as to facilitate their independence and self-care. These 10 key concepts convey IC, which is grounded in the personal and professional qualities of the care providers. These qualities include being loving, kind, patient, genuine, competent, helpful, consistent, and compassionate. IC also makes conceptual links between care, persons, the environment, and health. It is the result of blended understanding of the empirical, aesthetic, ethical, and intuitive aspects of an individual's life setting. An intersection of conditions, such as the skill of the care provider who supplies the key components of IC theory, results in a caring/nursing/healing relationship between the care providers and care recipients. This caring relationship subsequently ignites self-esteem and a sense of self-worth in the patient, which triggers motivation and empowerment for rediscovery of self and meaning in life. The end result is the patient's ability to manage daily life and participate in maintaining his or her own health.

Relationship of the Concept to Nursing and Health Research

In considering the relationship of IC theory to nursing and health research, particularly the field of mental health research, it proposes a qualitative research methodology for improving self-esteem and self-care (Kim, 1989). The empirical studies based on the IC model show that IC therapies have increased patients' self-esteem, motivated patients to undertake self-care more seriously, and helped them to improve social functioning (Kim et al., 1998; Kim, 2002; Kim & Kim, 2007a, 2007b; Min, Kim, So, & Joo, 2007). Moreover, IC therapies are effective not only in improving self-care, interpersonal relationships, and social functions but also in reducing the frequency and duration of hospitalization.

Relationship to Nursing Education

The interpersonal caring theory allows nursing students to apply its concepts in practice in the "real world." The simplicity and clarity of its 10 key components assist students in learning them and in applying them within their professional practice.

Relationship to Nursing Practice

Nurses' attentive listening to patients' stories and narrative pedagogy have only recently been recognized as a valid technique of teaching and learning (Gazarian, 2010). The narrative pedagogy, including storytelling in education, has been shown to be a method for teaching values and attitudes for professional development as well as enhancement of interpersonal and interprofessional communication. IC theory development is based on patients' stories or expression of their feelings toward wellness. The IC theory focuses on narratives from practice and studies that tell meaningful stories from patients' experiences in their own words. Thus, the theory is the retold stories of patients within a simple theoretical format that captures everyday examples of nursing practices.

SUMMARY

Based on Peplau's theory (1952, 1992) of interpersonal relations in nursing, Kim developed the IC theory that has been used in motivating patients to gain vitality and thus to achieve normalcy in their lives (Kim, 2012). The skillful administration of IC results in patients' building higher self-esteem. They gain creative energy through their nurses' loving and attentive caring. This IC theory includes 10 techniques: noticing, participating, sharing, active listening, companioning, complementing, comforting, hoping, forgiving, and accepting.

Studies have shown that the applications of this IC process results not only in patients' improving self-care, interpersonal relationships, and social functioning but also in achieving lower frequency and duration of institutionalization (Kim, 2002; Min et al., 2007). Moreover, this IC theory is relatively concrete for nurses to apply in diverse nursing education programs and practice settings. It is easy to teach and learn. Hence, it has a strong potential to guide nursing practice, education, and research.

REFERENCES

Gazarian, P. K. (2010). Digital stories: Incorporating narrative pedagogy. *Journal of Nursing Education, 49*, 287–290.

Kim, S. (1989). *Lived experiences of long-term psychiatric patients.* Annual conference proceedings, Research Institute of Nursing Science, Ewha Womans University, Seoul, South Korea.

Kim, S. (1997). *Effect of community-based psychiatric and mental health nursing in Korea.* Proceedings of International Conference on Interpersonal Relationships in Community-Based Mental Health Nursing, 95–107.

Kim, S. (2000). *Interpersonal caring: An intervention of improved self-esteem of long-term psychiatric patients in community.* Annual conference proceedings, Research Institute of Nursing Science, Ewha Womans University, Seoul, South Korea.

Kim, S. (2002). Interpersonal techniques: Concepts and quasi-experimental research. In H. Kashima, I. R. H. Falloon, M. Mizuno, & M. Asai (Eds.), *Comprehensive treatment of schizophrenia.* Tokyo: Springer.

Kim, S. (2012). *Interpersonal caring.* Seoul, South Korea: Soomoonsa.

Kim, S., & Ae, J. H. (1999). *Final report of UNDP supported project: Community-based mental health nursing program for rehabilitation of long-term psychiatric patients.* Research Institute of Nursing Science, Ewha Womans University, Seoul, South Korea.

Kim, S., & Berry, D. (1997). *Care for long-term psychiatric patients: A community based nursing model*. Proceedings of International Conference on Interpersonal Relationships in Community-Based Mental Health Nursing, 85–94.

Kim, S., & Kim, S. (2007a). Interpersonal caring: A theory for improved self-esteem in patients with long-term serious mental illness—I. *Asian Nursing Research, 1*, 11–22.

Kim, S., & Kim, S. (2007b). Interpersonal caring theory: An empirical test of its effectiveness utilizing growth curve analysis –II. *Asian Nursing Research, 1*, 187–198.

Kim, S., Kim, Y. H., Yang, S., Won, J. S., Lee, K. J., Lee, J. S., et al. (1998). Effect of interpersonal caring for homebound long-term psychiatric patients. *Korean Journal of Nursing Query, 7*, 100–124.

Kim, S., Lee, K., Lee, P., & Yang, S. (1997). Development of community-based psychiatric rehabilitation program. *Journal of Psychiatric-Mental Health Nursing, 6*, 5–19.

Min, S., Kim, S., So, H. S., & Joo, A. R. (2007). An effect of short-term interpersonal caring techniques to elderly women's grief and loneliness. *International Journal of Welfare for the Aged, 16*, 31–56.

Peplau, H. E. (1952). *Interpersonal Relations in Nursing*. New York, NY: Putnam.

Peplau, H. E. (1992). Interpersonal relations: A theoretical framework for application in nursing practice. *Nursing Science Quarterly, 5*, 13–18.

Travelbee, J. (1971). *Interpersonal Aspects of Nursing*. Philadelphia: F. A. Davis.

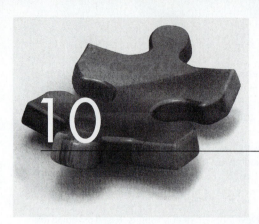

United Kingdom: The Person-Centered Nursing Model

Brendon McCormack and Tanya McCance

INTRODUCTION

Person-centeredness is a term that is becoming increasingly familiar within health and social care at a global level. It is being used to describe a standard of care that ensures that the patient is at the center of care delivery. Person-centered care has a long association with nursing and at the level of principle, is well understood as that which is concerned with treating a person as an individual, respecting the person's rights as a person, building mutual trust and understanding, and developing therapeutic relationships. Nurses have the expectation that people should receive a standard of care that reflects these principles. The inherent good of providing care within a philosophy of person-centeredness is irrefutable, but it has been recognized that translating the core concepts into every day practice is challenging. The reasons for this come in many forms and indicate the context in which care is being delivered and the fact that people are living in times of constant change, particularly within health and social care (McCormack & McCance, 2010).

The body of evidence relating to person-centered care is growing and with it there is increasing academic debate and critical dialogue regarding developments in this field. The main focus of attention in the current literature is the development of person-centeredness in practice and the strategies required to overcome the cultural and contextual challenges to implementing a person-centered approach (McCormack, Dewing, & McCance, 2011). Significantly, this agenda is being further fueled, particularly in the United Kingdom, by the increasing media reports of failures in care delivery resulting in a poor experience for patients, families, and staff (Berwick Report, 2013; Francis Report, 2013). In addition, there have been significant conceptual and theoretical advancements in the area of person-centeredness with the development of frameworks such as authentic consciousness (McCormack, 2003), the senses (Nolan, 2001), and the person-centered nursing (McCormack & McCance, 2010, 2006). The application and testing of these frameworks in practice (McCance, Gribben, McCormack, & Laird, 2013; McCormack, Karlsson, Dewing, & Lerdal, 2010; Ryan, Nolan, Reid, & Enderby, 2008) have gone some way in enhancing the understanding of how to effectively operationalize person-centeredness in practice. The focus of this chapter is on the person-centered nursing framework and its relevance to nursing practice.

BASIC ELEMENTS OF THE MODEL

The person-centered nursing framework was developed for use in the intervention stage of a large quasiexperimental project that focused on measuring the effectiveness of the implementation of person-centered nursing in a tertiary hospital setting (McCormack et al. 2008). The framework was derived from McCormack's conceptual framework (McCormack, 2001, 2003) focusing on person-centered practice with older people and McCance's framework (2003) focusing on patients' and nurses' experience of care in nursing. These two conceptual frameworks were selected for the following reasons:

- Both were derived from a humanistic perspective of caring.
- An initial review of the frameworks indicated a high degree of consistency across individual concepts and thus a high degree of face validity.
- Both were derived from inductive and systematic collaborative research processes.
- Collectively, they represented a synthesis of the then available literature on caring and person-centeredness.

A systematic process was used in the development of the original person-centered nursing framework and continues to evolve through extensive testing in research, education, and practice (McCormack & McCance, 2006).

Before describing the framework in detail, it is important to place it on the continuum of theory development. This is done by drawing on the seminal work of Fawcett (1995), who describes a hierarchy of nursing knowledge that has five components. At the highest level of abstraction is the *metaparadigm* that represents a broad consensus for nursing and provides general parameters for the field; next to this are *philosophies*, which provide a statement of beliefs and values. *Conceptual models* are at the next level and provide a particular frame of reference that says something about "how to observe and interpret the phenomena of interest to the discipline" (Fawcett, 3). *Theories*, which are less abstract than conceptual models, are the third component in the hierarchy. They can be further described as grand theories or middle-range theories, with the latter being narrower in scope and "made up of concepts and propositions that are empirically measurable" (Fawcett, 25). Fawcett distinguishes between conceptual models and mid-range theories in that mid-range theories articulate one or more relatively concrete and specific concepts that are derived from a conceptual model. Furthermore, the propositions that describe these concepts propose specific relationships among them. The final component in the hierarchy of nursing knowledge is the *empirical indicator*, which provides the means of measuring concepts within a middle-range theory. The person-centered nursing framework has been described as a middle-range theory in that it has been derived from two abstract conceptual frameworks, comprises concepts that are relatively specific, and outlines relationships among the concepts. The following sections describe the concepts within the framework and how they relate, thus demonstrating its value as a middle-range theory.

Key Concepts of the Model/Theory

The person-centered nursing framework essentially comprises four constructs: *prerequisites* that focus on the attributes of the nurse, *the care environment* that focuses on the context in which care is delivered, *person-centered processes* that focus on delivering care through a range of activities, and *expected outcomes* that are the results of effective person-centered nursing. The relationship among the constructs of the framework is indicated by the pictorial representation: Being able to reach the center of the framework, the prerequisites must first be considered and then the care environment, which is necessary in providing effective care through the care processes. This ordering ultimately leads to the achievement of the outcomes: the central component of the framework. It is also acknowledged that there are relationships within and across constructs.

The Prerequisites.   The *prerequisites* focus on the attributes of the nurse and include being professionally competent, having developed interpersonal skills, being committed to the job, being able to demonstrate clarity of beliefs and values, and knowing self. Professional competence focuses on the knowledge and skills of the nurse to make decisions and prioritize care, and it includes competence in relation to physical or technical aspects of care. Having highly developed interpersonal skills reflects the nurse's ability to communicate at a variety of levels. Commitment to the job indicates the dedication of nurses and the sense that they want to provide care that is best for the patient. Clarity of beliefs and values highlights the importance of the nurse knowing his or her own views and being aware of how he or she can impact decisions made by the patient. This is closely linked to knowing self and the assumption that before being able to help others, a nurse needs to have insight into how he or she functions as a person. See Table 10–1 for the definitions used for each of these components.

The Care Environment.   The *care environment* focuses on the context in which care is delivered and includes appropriate skill mix, systems that facilitate shared decision making power, effective staff relationships, supportive organizational systems, and potential for innovation and risk taking. Appropriate skill mix highlights the potential impact of staffing levels on the delivery of effective person-centered care and emphasizes the importance of the composition of the team in achieving positive outcomes for patients. Shared decision making depends on having in place systems and processes that facilitate a dialogue among those involved in the caring interaction. This can include the patient, family member, caregiver or nurse, doctor, or other health professional. Shared decision making is

TABLE 10–1   Definitions of the Prerequisites

Professionally competent: The knowledge, skills, and attitudes of the practitioner to negotiate care options and effectively provide holistic care.

Developed interpersonal skills: The ability of the practitioner to communicate at a variety of levels with others using effective verbal and nonverbal interactions that show personal concern for others' situations and a commitment to finding mutual solutions.

Commitment to job: The dedication of individuals and team members demonstrated to patients, families, and communities through intentional engagement that focuses on providing holistic evidence-informed care.

Knowing 'self': The way an individual makes sense of her or his knowing, being, and becoming a person-centered practitioner through reflection, self-awareness, and engagement with others.

Clarity of beliefs and values: The awareness of the impact of beliefs and values on care provided by practitioners and received by service users and the commitment to reconcile beliefs and values in ways that facilitate person-centeredness.

---

also closely linked to the development of effective staff relationships and to the sharing of power. It is important, however, to note that the sharing of power also relates to the power base between the patient and the nurse, which reflects one of the basic tenants of person-centeredness described earlier. The identification of supportive organizational systems acknowledges the incredible influence that organizational culture can have on the quality of care delivered and the freedom afforded to practitioners to work autonomously, reflecting the potential for innovation and risk taking. The care environment and the components described here have a significant impact on the operationalization of person-centered nursing and have the greatest potential to limit or enhance its facilitation (McCormack, 2004). This is consistent with a contemporary view of using knowledge in practice in which the context of practice is recognized as having a highly significant impact on clinical effectiveness. Refer to Table 10–2 for the definition of each of these components.

Person-Centered Processes. *Person-centered processes* focus on delivering care through a range of activities that operationalize person-centered nursing and include working with patient's beliefs and values, engagement, having sympathetic presence, sharing decision making, and providing holistic care. This is the component of the framework that

TABLE 10–2   Definitions of Components within the Care Environment

Skill mix: Most often considered from a nursing context, this refers to the ratio of registered nurses (RNs) and nonregistered nurses in a ward or unit nursing team; in a multidisciplinary context is the range of staff with the requisite knowledge and skills needed to provide a quality service.

Shared decision-making systems: Methods that facilitate active participation in decision making by all team members.

Effective staff relationships: Interpersonal connections that are productive in the achievement of holistic person-centered care.

Power sharing: Nondominant, nonhierarchical relationship that does not exploit individuals but is concerned with achieving the best mutually accepted outcomes through agreed values, goals, wishes, and desires.

Potential for innovation and risk taking: Capability to exercise professional accountability in decision making that reflects a balance between the best available evidence, professional judgment, local information, and patient/family preferences.

Physical environment: Health care setting that balances aesthetics with function by paying attention to design, dignity, privacy, sanctuary, choice/control, safety, and universal access with the intention of improving patient, family, and staff operational performance and outcomes (adapted from Hospice friendly Hospitals Programme http://hospicefoundation.ie/healthcare-programmes/hospice-friendly-hospitals/initiatives-staff-development/design-dignity/design-dignity/ accessed 4/02/2015).

Supportive organizational systems: Methods that promote initiative, creativity, freedom, and safety of persons underpinned by a governance framework that emphasizes culture, relationships, values, communication, professional autonomy, and accountability.

specifically focuses on the patient; it describes person-centered nursing in the context of care delivery. Working with patients' beliefs and values reinforces one of the fundamental principles of person-centered nursing, which places importance on developing a clear picture of what the patient values about his or her life and how he or she makes sense of what is happening. This is closely linked to shared decision making, which focuses on nurses' facilitating patient participation by providing information and integrating newly formed perspectives into established practices. It Shared decision-making depends, however, on systems that facilitate this making (the care environment). This environment must support processes of negotiation that consider individual values to form a legitimate basis for decision making, the achievement of which rests on successful processes of communication. Having sympathetic presence highlights an engagement that recognizes the uniqueness and value of the individual and reflects the quality of the nurse–patient relationship. Finally, providing holistic care focuses not only on providing physical care but also on meeting the spiritual and psychosocial needs of patients and their families. See Table 10–3 for the definitions used for each of these components.

The Expected Outcomes

The term *expected outcomes* refers to the central construct of the framework and the results expected from effective person-centered nursing. The outcomes include experience of good care, involvement in care, feeling of well-being, and creation of a healthful environment. The experience of good care reflects the evaluation that a patient, or indeed a nurse, places on her or his care experience. Involvement in care is the outcome expected as

TABLE 10–3 Definitions of the Person-Centered Processes

Working with patient's beliefs and values: Clearly understanding what the patient values about his or her life and how he or she makes sense of what is happening from his or her individual perspective, psychosocial context, and social role.

Shared Decision-making: Being involved in the decision making of patients and others significant to them by considering values, experiences, concerns, and future aspirations.

Engagement: The practitioner's being connected with a patient and others significant to the patient determined by knowledge of the person, clarity of beliefs and values, knowledge of self, and professional expertise.

Providing holistic care: Delivering treatment and care that pays attention to the whole person through the integration of physiological, psychological, sociocultural, developmental, and spiritual dimensions of persons.

Having sympathetic presence: Being engaged by recognizing the uniqueness and value of the individual by appropriately responding to cues that maximize coping resources through the recognition of important agendas in the person's life.

a result of participating in shared decision-making processes, and a feeling of well-being indicates a sense of being valued. Creation of a therapeutic environment is described as one in which decision making is shared, staff relationships are collaborative, leadership is transformational, and innovative practices are supported; it is the ultimate outcome for teams working to develop a person-centered workplace.

RELATIONSHIP OF THE FRAMEWORK TO CONCEPTS INHERENT IN THE METAPARADIGM OF NURSING

The utility of the person-centered nursing framework to nursing practice is reinforced by the way it aligns with the concepts inherent within the metaparadigm of nursing, namely the concepts of nursing, person, health, and environment.

Definition and Description of Nursing

The essence of nursing depicted within the person-centered nursing framework reflects the ideals of humanistic caring in which there is a moral component, and practice has at its basis a therapeutic intent, which is translated through relationships that are built on effective interpersonal processes. Therefore, person-centeredness in nursing practice requires the formation of therapeutic relationships among professionals, patients, and others significant to them in their lives and the building of these relationships are based on mutual trust, understanding, and sharing collective knowledge (McCormack, 2001; Dewing, 2004; Binnie & Titchen 1999). The definition used within the framework was developed in a national nursing action research program in Ireland, which closely reflects this literature and is consistent with the understandings of person-centeredness within a nursing context (McCormack et al., 2010b, 1):

> Person-centeredness is an approach to practice established through the formation and fostering of therapeutic relationships between all care providers, older people and others significant to them in their lives. It is underpinned by values of respect for persons, individual right to self determination, mutual respect and understanding. It is enabled by cultures of empowerment that foster continuous approaches to practice development.

The framework highlights the complexity of person-centered nursing, and through the articulation of the key constructs, emphasizes the contextual, attitudinal, and moral dimensions of humanistic caring practices. The relationship between the constructs describes the necessity for competent nurses who have the ability to manage the numerous contextual and attitudinal factors that exist within care environments and to engage in processes that keep the person at the center of caring interactions.

Definition and Description of Person

The concept of person is central to the person-centered nursing framework and captures those attributes that represent our humanness and the way in which people construct their lives. How they think about moral values; how they express political, spiritual, or religious beliefs; and how they engage emotionally and in their relationships and the kind of lives they want to live are all shaped by their attributes as persons. How the concept of persons is defined within the framework draws on the early work of Kitwood (1997, 8) who defined person-centeredness as "a standing or status that is bestowed upon one human being by others, in the context of relationship and social being. It implies recognition, respect and trust."

Furthermore, the framework is underpinned by four different perspectives on the concept of person, each providing a different lens that ultimately shapes the way person-centeredness is operationalized in practice. *Being in relation* emphasizes the importance of relationships and the interpersonal processes that enable the development of relationships that have therapeutic benefit. *Being in a social world* considers persons to be interconnected with their social world, creating and recreating meaning through their being in the world. Closely linked to being in a social world is *being with self*, which emphasizes the importance of persons' "knowing self" and the values they hold about their lives and how they make sense of what is happening to them. *Being in place* encourages people to pay attention to "place" recognizing the impact of the "milieu of care" on the care experience. These perspectives are not mutually exclusive and in the real world, people do not think about themselves and others being in this fragmented way. No one position stands alone when thinking about decision making in practice. The reality is that people might have to draw from all these perspectives in order to make informed person-centered decisions. One way to enable such integration to happen is through being authentic, and, according to Gadow (1980, 85) is "a way of reaching decisions which are truly one's own—decisions that express all that one believes important about oneself and the world, the entire complexity of one's values." This description of person is central to the framework and requires nurses to have the ability to facilitate an individual's authenticity, so that his or her full potential can be realized and his or her capacity to exercise autonomous action maximized, despite the constraining factors that can exist in the environment.

Definition and Description of Environment

Within the framework, *creating a therapeutic culture* reflects the extent to which the environment supports and maintains person-centered principles and is described as one in which decision making is shared, staff relationships are collaborative, leadership is transformational, and innovative practices are supported. McCormack et al. (2011) suggest that contextual factors, such as organizational culture, the learning environment, and the care environment itself, pose the greatest challenge to person-centeredness and the development of cultures that can sustain person-centered care. Further research by Brown and McCormack (2011) brought into stark focus the impact of the environment of care on evidence-informed person-centered practice. Brown and McCormack studied postoperative pain management practices with older people following abdominal surgery. The researchers found that barriers to effective postoperative pain management did not depend on which decision-making tools were used (such as algorithms and protocols) but had more to do with the "psychological safety" of the care environment. A psychologically safe care environment is one in which staff feel safe to give and receive feedback about their practice, where leadership facilitates open and honest dialogue, and where the culture supports reflection on practice. This type of practice culture is consistent with person-centered values and, the researchers suggest, is critical to practicing person-centered nursing.

The built environment also has an impact on the effectiveness of person-centered nursing. Good design directly impacts quality of life (Callaghan, Netten, & Darton, 2009), and it is likely that the design of care facilities has an effect on the well-being of patients and staff. For example, a long-term care facility that has communal areas that are welcoming and accessible by all encourages social interaction; people can meet or have group activities. Having quiet spaces is an equally important component of quality of life, providing for reflection and stillness. A care environment with a calming atmosphere that uses music, lighting, and soft furnishings facilitates reading or reflection. The challenge is to ensure that busy health care facilities are also sensitive and responsive to well-being, both physical and emotional.

Definition and Description of Health

Within the person-centered nursing framework is a broader notion of health that reflects living a positive life, which embraces all dimensions of being. Considering a social model of health, the authors have focused on the work of Seedhouse (1986) who refers to a set of conditions that enables a person to work to reach his or her potential and describes health in relation to "foundations for achievement." The foundations that make up health, according to Seedhouse, include the basic needs of food, drink, shelter, warmth and so on; access to the widest possible information and the skills and confidence to assimilate this information; and the recognition that an individual is never totally isolated from other people and the external environment and cannot be fully understood separated from the influence of his or her environment. This broader notion of health reflects a therapeutic environment from the perspective of staff as one in which they are supported and enabled to deliver person-centered care in line with their values. This conceptualization is also supported by work undertaken by Titchen and McCormack on enabling human flourishing (McCormack & Titchen, 2006; Titchen & McCormack, 2010). These authors argue that human flourishing is the overall outcome arising from working in a person-centered way. They argue that when practitioners integrate the creative energies of different forms of knowledge and intelligences, growthful experiences for all (staff, service users, families, for example) are enabled.

ANALYSIS AND EVALUATION

Relationship to Nursing and Health Research

Since its publication, the person-centered nursing framework has been used to structure implementation studies that focused on the development of person-centered nursing in a variety of practice settings. Through the use of the framework in this way, relationships between concepts have been identified and refined and led to the development of new areas of research. Implementation studies have been undertaken in residential care settings for older people, in a variety of secondary and tertiary care settings, in community care, and in palliative care (McCance et al., 2013; McCormack et al., 2010b; Brown & McCormack, 2011). These studies used the framework to promote an increased understanding of person-centered nursing with the aim of enabling practitioners to recognize key elements in their practice, generate meaning from data that can inform the development of person-centered nursing, and, most importantly, focus the implementation and evaluation of developments in practice; see, for example, the Essentials of Care Program in NSW, Australia (http://www.health.nsw.gov.au/nursing/projects/Pages/eoc.aspx) accessed August 2014. Furthermore, there is evidence of the international adoption of the framework in research and development in, for example, Canada (Cowie & Janes, 2011). There has also been significant development of a range of tools that enable the evaluation of the relationship between a person-centered approach to nursing and the resulting outcomes for patients and nurses (McCormack et al., 2010a; Slater & McCormack, 2007). There is, however, still much to be achieved in the area of outcome evaluation with current research focusing on the development of an outcomes framework. This builds on the components in the outcomes construct of the person-centered nursing framework (McCormack, McCance, & Maben, 2013).

Relationship to Nursing Education

There are various styles and approaches to learning, but being able to respond to them in different learning situations is challenging, particularly if the goal is to embrace concepts of person-centeredness in the curriculum. Globally, nursing education curricula have been challenged to respond to contemporary health and care agendas, such as patient safety, self-management, expanding and extending roles, and, of course, a shift to more person-centered orientations in service delivery and care management. The need for educators to develop and extend existing modes of learning in order to advance these agendas and develop person-centered nurses is essential. If the ultimate outcome is to produce a nurse who can creatively solve a problem or plan an innovative care intervention for their patients, then it follows that educators have a responsibility to nurture students' creative capacity in order to respond effectively in a person-centered way. Being able to trust learners to work with their own ways of thinking through problems, challenges, and situations is a core skill in adult learning (Knowles, 1984). Knowles demonstrated the differences that exist between adult learners and children (what Knowles referred to as the differences between andragogy and pedagogy) with a critical element of this being the need to understand how adults process information. Unlike the "rotelike" and repetitive approach to learning usually adopted for children, adults tend to learn through connections, images, metaphors, and meanings. Therefore, developing curricula that enhance the creative capacity of nursing students is essential in the development of person-centered practices. The foundation of such a curriculum lies in the concept of "knowing self" in the person-centered nursing framework. Knowing self is critical to being a reflexive practitioner: Knowing when a person is being authentic, knowing when the person is being challenged, knowing the person's dislikes, and so on are all aspects of knowing that are essential to nurses engaging in an authentic and person-centered way with patients and colleagues. The authors of this chapter believe that knowing self requires educators to be creative in their approaches to exploring "self" in order to provoke new understandings about self and the ways in which this knowing helps people to be more person centered.

Learning how to let go of control and enable students to take risks is also essential for nurses to learn how to work with patient's beliefs and values and their individually expressed needs. The need for educators to be in control has been identified in the educational research literature (Greene, 2007); indeed, in the world of education action research, there is often an emphasis in "first-person action research" (Burgess, 2006) on helping educators to release control over learning to learners. Nursing curricula need to embrace risk taking as a key focus that enables students to develop the prerequisites for being person-centered nurses.

Relationship to Professional Practice

The fundamental use of the person-centered nursing framework is as a tool to enable the operationalization of person-centered nursing in practice. It has been used to promote an increased understanding of person-centered care with the aim of enabling practitioners to recognize key elements in their practice. It also has been used as an analytical framework to generate meaning from data that can inform the development of person-centered practice. Most importantly, however, it has been used as a tool that can assist practitioners to identify barriers to change and to focus the implementation and evaluation of developments in practice. It has been argued that the promotion of person-centered cultures has the capacity to make a critical difference to the care experience of patients and staff (McCance et al., 2013; McCormack et al., 2008; McCormack et al., 2010c). Whereas organizations might aspire to a standard of care that reflects these components, the reality of the quality of care delivered can often be something different. This brings to the fore the need to focus on attitudes, behaviors, and relationships and reflects the importance of engaging in new ways of thinking and working that promote a person-centered approach. The application of the person-centered nursing framework by individuals and teams has the potential to contribute to clarifying the attitudes and behaviors necessary for good quality nursing care, as well as the kind of relationships needed to nurture these essential attributes of professional practice. As described in this chapter, research to date has demonstrated the impact of person-centredness on professional practice.

SUMMARY

This chapter presents the person-centered nursing framework, a model that has been developed from practice for use in practice. The framework highlights the complexity of person-centered nursing, and, through the articulation of the key constructs, emphasizes the contextual, attitudinal, and moral dimensions of humanistic caring practices. The relationship between the constructs describe the necessity for competent nurses who have the ability to manage the numerous contextual and attitudinal factors that exist within care environments and to engage in processes that keep the person at the center of caring interactions. The outcomes arising from the development of person-centered practice demonstrates the potential to enhance the care experience for both patients and staff.

REFERENCES

Berwick Report. (2013). *A promise to learn—A commitment to act*. London: Stationery Office.

Binnie, A., & Titchen, A. (1999). *Freedom to practise: The development of patient-centred nursing*. Oxford, UK: Elsevier.

Brown, D., & McCormack, B. (2011). Developing the practice context to enable more effective pain management with older people: An action research approach. *Implementation Science, 6*(9), 1.

Burgess, J. (2006). Participatory action research: First-person perspectives of a graduate student. *Action Research, 4*, 419–437.

Callaghan, L., Netten, A., & Darton, R. (2009). *The development of social well-being in new extra care housing schemes*. York, UK: Joseph Rowntree Foundation.

Cowie, B. G., & Janes, N. (2011). Hip deep in the messy lowland: Using fourth generation evaluation to make sense of practice complexities. *International Practice Development Journal, 1*(2), article 8.

Dewing, J. (2004). Concerns relating to the application of frameworks to promote person-centredness in nursing with older people. *International Journal of Older People Nursing, 13*(3a), 39–44.

Fawcett, J. (1995). *Analysis and evaluation of conceptual models of nursing* (3rd ed.). Philadelphia: F. A. Davis.

Francis Report. (2013). *Report of the Mid Staffordshire NHS Foundation Trust public inquiry*. London: Stationary Office.

Gadow, S. (1980). Existential advocacy: Philosophical foundations of nursing. In S. F. Spicker & S. Gadow (Eds.), *Nursing: Images and ideals—Opening dialogue with the humanities*. New York: Springer.

Greene, D. (2007). Gatekeepers: The role of adult education practitioners and programs in social control. *Journal for Critical Education Policy Studies, 5*(2), 2. http://www.jceps.com/print.php?articleID=107

Kitwood, T. (1997). *Dementia reconsidered: The person comes first*. Milton Keynes, Bedfordshire: Open University Press.

Knowles, M. (1984). *The adult learner: A neglected species* (3rd ed.). Houston: Gulf Publishing.

McCance, T. V. (2003). Caring in nursing practice: The development of a conceptual framework. *Research and Theory for Nursing Practice: An International Journal, 17*(2), 101–116.

McCance, T., Gribben, B., McCormack, B., & Laird, E. (2013). Promoting person-centred practice within acute care: The impact of culture and context on a facilitated practice development programme. *International Practice Development Journal, 3*(1), 2.

McCormack, B. (2001). *Negotiating partnerships with older people—A person-centred approach.* Basingstoke, UK: Ashgate.

McCormack, B. (2003). A conceptual framework for person-centred practice with older people. *International Journal of Nursing Practice, 9,* 202–209.

McCormack, B. (2004). Person-centredness in gerontological nursing: An overview of the literature. *Journal of Clinical Nursing, 13*(3a), 31–38.

McCormack, B., Dewing, J., Breslin, E., Coyne-Nevin, A., Kennedy, K., Manning, M., and Slater, P. (2010a). Developing person-centred practice: Nursing outcomes arising from changes to the care environment in residential settings for older people. *International Journal of Older People Nursing, 5,* 93–107.

McCormack, B., Dewing, J., Breslin, L., Tobin, C., Manning, M., Coyne-Nevin, A., & Peelo-Kilroe, L. (2010b). The implementation of a model of person-centred practice in older person settings: Final report. Dublin, Ireland: Office of the Nursing Services Director, Health Services Executive.

McCormack, B., Dewing, J., & McCance, T. (2011). Developing person-centred care: Addressing contextual challenges through practice development. *Online Journal of Issues in Nursing, 16*(2), 3.

McCormack, B., Karlsson, B., Dewing, J., & Lerdal, A. (2010c). Exploring person-centredness: A qualitative meta-synthesis of four studies. *Scandinavian Journal of Caring Sciences, 24,* 620–634.

McCormack, B., & McCance T. (2006) Development of a framework for person-centred nursing. *Journal of Advanced Nursing, 56*(5): 1–8.

McCormack, B., & McCance, T. V. (2010). *Person-centred nursing: Theory and practice.* Oxford, UK: Wiley Blackwell.

McCormack, B., McCance, T. V., & Maben J. (2013). Outcome evaluation in the development of person-centred practice. In B. McCormack, K. Manley, & A. Titchen (Eds.), *Practice development in nursing and healthcare* (pp. 190–211). Oxford, UK: Wiley-Blackwell.

McCormack, B., McCance, T. V., Slater, P., McCormick, J., McArdle, C., & Dewing, J. (2008). Person-centred outcomes and cultural change. In K. Manley, B. McCormack, & V. Wilson (Eds.), *International practice development in nursing and healthcare* (pp. 189–214). Oxford, UK: Blackwell.

McCormack, B., & Titchen, A. (2006). Critical creativity: Melding, exploding, blending. *Educational Action Research, 14*(2), 239–266.

Nolan, M. (2001) Successful ageing: Keeping the 'person' in person-centred care. *British Journal of Nursing, 10*(7), 450–454.

Ryan, T., Nolan, M., Reid, D., & Enderby, P. (2008). Using the senses framework to achieve relationship centred dementia care services. *Dementia, 7*(1), 71–93.

Seedhouse, D. (1986). *Health: The foundations for achievement.* London: Wiley.

Slater, P., & McCormack, B. (2007). An exploration of the factor structure of the Nursing Work Index. *Worldviews on Evidence-Based Nursing, 4*(1), 30–39.

Titchen, A., & McCormack, B. (2010). Dancing with stones: Critical creativity as methodology for human flourishing. *Educational Action Research, 18*(4), 531–554.

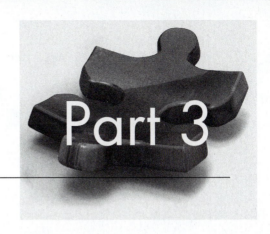

Part 3

Applications of U.S.-Developed Nursing Models to Nursing in Other Countries

CHAPTER OUTLINE

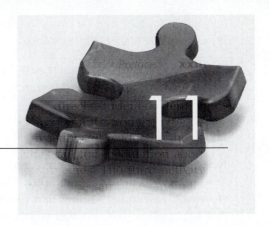

Egypt: Applications of Nursing Theory

*Zeinab Ahmed, Moukhtar Abdelsalam,
and Naglaa Mostafa Gaber*

INTRODUCTION

The commitment to nursing as a profession and career is based on solid grounds that come from the use of nursing theories and models and evidence-based research and practices. The increasing use of nursing theories in all aspects of nursing has contributed to enhancing nursing as a profession and helped many nurses around the world to develop their careers. In addition, the use of nursing theories and evidence-based practice have attributed to the development of many recent nursing specialties around the globe.

In developing countries, the use of nursing theories is still developing and has minimal or no obvious impact on nursing education and practice. A thorough investigation of nursing theories has in Egypt was performed to collect the relevant data for this chapter. It found that in nursing education and practice, the use of nursing theories is very limited and are available only in postgraduate students programs (master's and doctoral). In Egypt, although many nursing faculties are teaching courses related to theory development and application specifically in doctoral programs, a very limited number of students use nursing theories as guides for their dissertations and theses. The reasons for this could be related to the nature of the study or a lack of available guidance on how to use nursing theory as a guide for a research study.

Nevertheless, this chapter will show how nursing theories are utilized in Egypt whether in nursing research, education, or practice.

NURSING RESEARCH

Research on the use of nursing theories in Egypt has been done primarily by doctoral students mostly at the Cairo University Faculty of Nursing. However, researchers found that few nursing theories are employed in a real-life applications; in other words, a national generalization of research findings is lacking.

In the past 10 years, however, doctoral candidates in nursing studies in Egypt have used different nursing theories as guides for their dissertations. For example, Abdelsalam (2011) studied the effect of supportive psychotherapy on interpersonal relationships, personality pathology, and social adjustment among hospitalized women who were depressed. These candidates used both Peplau's interpersonal model and Roy's adaptation model in their studies.

Integration of the Models in the Study

According to Abdelsalam (2011), Peplau's theory (1991) focuses on the interpersonal processes and therapeutic relationship that develops between the nurse and client. The interpersonal focus requires the nurse to attend to the interpersonal processes that occur between the nurse and patient. The interpersonal process is a maturing force for personality. Interpersonal processes include the nurse–patient relationship, communication, pattern integration, and the roles of the nurse. *Psychodynamic nursing* is defined as being able to understand one's own behavior to help others identify the difficulties they feel and apply principles of human relations to the problems that arise at all levels of experience. This theory stresses the importance of nurses' ability to understand their own behavior in order to help others identify perceived difficulties.

This study was guided by Sister Roy's adaptation model (RAM) in examining the effects of supportive psychotherapy (SP) on interpersonal problems, personality pathology, and social adjustment among depressed women who were hospitalized. The broad nature of RAM, developed by Roy, allows an examination of SP and the development of a theory-based intervention from an expanded, integrated, and holistic nursing perspective. According to RAM, human beings and groups are perceived as biopsychosocial adaptive systems that hold a set of related units having inputs of control and feedback processes and outputs that constantly change and interact with their environment. Health is a process of being and becoming integrated and whole and reflects both the environment and the person. The control processes are coping mechanisms manifested by four adaptive modes including physiologic, self-concept, role function, and interdependence. More specifically, the person is defined asan adaptive system with cognator and regulator processes acting to maintain adaptation in four adaptive modes (Fitzpatrick & Whall, 2005).

Accordingly, the key concepts of Roy's model were integrated with Abdelsalam's (2011) study variables: the individual as a biopsychosocial being, the four adaptive modes, the regulator and cognator coping processes, and behavior responses.

Concepts of the Abdelsalam's Derived Model

Biopsychosocial Being.   The RAM model depicts the individual as a biopsychosocial being who is able to adapt to environmental stimuli categorized as focal, contextual, or residual. In assessing the physical domain, depression is viewed as the focal stimulus that leads to maladaptive responses in women. The contextual stimuli are indirectly related to the focal stimuli, such as the patient's personality pathology. The residual stimuli are all other stimuli that affect the focal and contextual stimuli, such as interpersonal problems with family and friends, social adjustment in domains such as performing daily living activities independently, and the ability to interact in social situations such as group work and recreational activities.

Adaptive Modes.   According to RAM, adaptation is assessed and measured in physical (physiologic) and psychosocial (self-concept, role function, and interdependence) modes. The physiologic mode is the sum of all physical and chemical processes involved in a living organism's functions and activities. There is an important and accumulating body of evidence to indicate that the physical consequences of depression are far from benign. In particular, the consequences included the increased risk of coronary artery disease and the impact on bone mineral content, both of which have received recent attention as a result from depression (Porter, Linsley, & Ferrier, 2001). Patients with depression usually experience difficulty with physical activities; their energy levels are usually reduced; and their sense of personal health is adversely affected, as are their abilities to interact socially, to work effectively, and to manage their homes (Kennedy, Eisfeld, Hons, & Cooke, 2001). Specifically, the Abdelsalam (2011) study found that depression assessment represented the physiologic mode as illustrated in Figure (11–1).

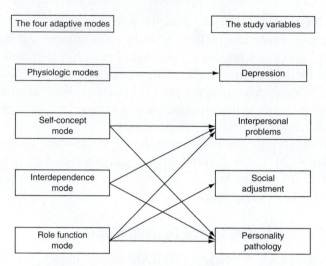

FIGURE 11–1   Integration of Adaptive Modes
and the Study Variables.

The self-concept mode is the composite of the beliefs and feelings an individual possesses about herself or himself at a given time. Having one's self-esteem depend on a given domain such as relationships with others is termed "contingent self-esteem" and was conceptualized early James (1890). According to contingency of self-worth models, people differ according to the domains on which they base their self-worth, (Crocker & Park, 2004; Croker & Wolfe, 2001). One domain in which one's self-esteem can be contingent is that of interpersonal relationships with others. According to RAM, the interdependence adaptive mode refers to giving and receiving love via nurturing relationships. Therefore, when a person has an underdeveloped social network, she or he will not be able to handle the pressures of an individual life, and a negatively framed social network can actually reinforce thoughts of hopelessness, failure, and being worthless. Therefore, Abdelsalam (2011) used interpersonal problems to represent both the self-concept and the interdependence adaptive modes.

The *role function mode* is a set of expectations about how a person functions and relates with others. Consequences of Major Depressive Disorder (MDD) exceed personal distress to include significant psychosocial dysfunction in domains such as work, family and social relationships, and leisure activities Abdelsalam (2011) integrated social adjustment and interpersonal problems to represent the role function mode. Finally, personality pathology in the current study represents the self-concept, interdependence, and role function modes as shown in Figure (11–1).

Regulator and Cognator Coping Processes

The regulator and cognator subsystems are the mechanisms for adapting to or coping with a changing environment and are viewed as biological, psychological, and social in origin. They are both innate and acquired; some mechanisms are genetically determined or common to the species whereas other mechanisms are acquired through processes such as learning. The regulator subsystem responds through neural, chemical, and endocrine channels whereas the cognator subsystem responds through cognitive-emotive channels. These channels include perceptual information for processing, learning, judgment, and emotion, which include defenses to seek relief. These responses of regulator and cognator subsystems are manifested or carried out through the four effectors' modes (Fitzpatrick & Whall, 2005). In the Abdelsalam (2011) study, the researcher performed SP to enhance patients' regulator and cognator coping processes as explained by Figure (11–2).

For the regulator processes, the researcher used the free association technique to facilitate a patient's expression of feelings. Thus, the patient's emotions were explored and understood. Also, the researcher used stress management strategies to enhance the patient's neural, chemical, and endocrine functioning. The provision of physical care, such as regular bathing for the patients, also can enhance their regulator adaptation. Regarding the cognator processes, the researcher educated the patients about depression and its symptoms and management. Self-esteem enhancement strategies also were used.

Behavior Response.   *Behavior* is described as "all responses of the human adaptive system including capacities, assets, knowledge, skills, abilities, and commitments" (Fitzpatrick & Whall, 2005). Behavior includes both internal and external actions and reactions that are formulated as adaptive or ineffective responses. According to Roy and Andrews (1999), adaptive responses are those behaviors that promote the integrity of the human system whereas ineffective responses are those that neither promote integrity nor contribute to the adaptive processes of survival, growth, reproduction, or mastery.

Unit term: Hospitalized depressed Egyptian women

Time unit:

- *Time 1*: The point in time of assessing the patient's biopsychosocial adaptation before engaging in the supportive psychotherapy program.
- *Time 2*: The point in time that refers to the behavior response expressed by depressed hospitalized women after participating in the supportive psychotherapy program as shown in Figure (11–2).

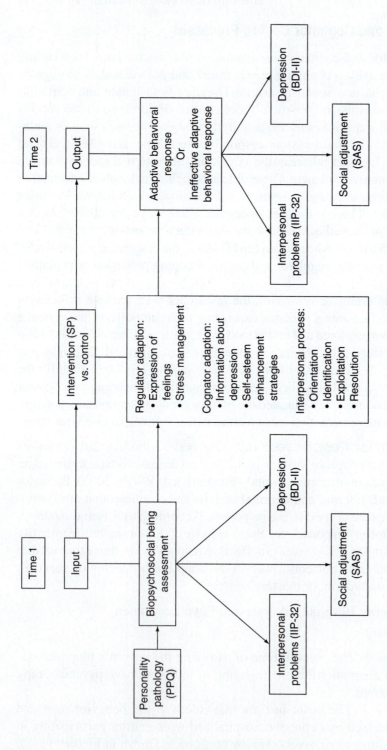

FIGURE 11–2 Proposed Model.

BDI: Beck depression inventory   PPQ: Personality pathology questionnaire
IIP-32: Inventory of interpersonal problems-32   SAS: Social adjustment scale

CONCEPTUAL DEFINITIONS OF THE STUDY'S MAJOR VARIABLES

RAM, Peplau, and Study Variables

George, Ellison, and Larson (2002) explained that RAM is based on the premise that humans are biopsychosocial beings and an individual's behavior is related to the behavior of others. Consequently, a person's external environment has a large impact on his or her well-being because he or she is always interacting with it. Accordingly, a person's ability to cope can be impeded by some external stressors. This is the point at which nurses should intervene to support patients as they deal with these stressors, thus promoting their overall health. Roy (1970) explained that the biopsychosocial being adapts through four modes of adaptation.

An individual first adapts to *physiologic needs* such as nutrition, rest, and exercise. The second mode of adaptation is the *self-concept* as determined by interactions with others. *Role function* indicates the mode used when individuals respond to their position in society. The final mode used to adapt is *interdependence*, which involves relationships neither dependent nor independent with others. Accordingly, Roy (1970) views nursing as a means of supporting an individual's adaptation in each of the four modes. Therefore Abdelsalam's (2011) assessment of the biopsychosocial being concept involves looking at a patient's depression, interpersonal problems, personality pathology, and social adjustment to indicate the four adaptive modes explained by RAM.

- Interpersonal problems are defined as individual or personal recurrent difficulties in relating to others (Locke, 2000). Utilizing RAM, interpersonal problems indicate the self-concept and interdependence adaptive modes. Accordingly, *interpersonal problem* is defined as the composite of the negative beliefs and feelings an individual possesses about himself or herself at a given time that result in problems of giving and receiving love and nurturing others. Interpersonal problems were measured using the Inventory of Interpersonal Problems-32 (IIP-32) (Barkham, Hardy, & Startup, 1996). It assesses domains of interpersonal relationships such as caring, openness, aggressiveness, assertiveness, supporting others, and dependence, which indicate the person's self-concept and interdependence.
- Personality pathology involves the enduring patterns of behavior and emotion that bring the person into repeated conflict with others or prevent the person from performing expected social and occupational roles (Pargament, Koenig, Tarakeshwar, & Hahn, 2004).

According to RAM, personality pathology indicates self-concept, interdependence, and role function adaptive modes. Accordingly, *personality pathology* is defined as the negative beliefs and feelings an individual possesses about himself or herself at a given time that result in problems of giving and receiving love and nurturing others, which leads to negative expectations about how a person functions and relates with others. Personality pathology is measured by means of the personality pathology questionnaire developed by the researcher and based on the Taylor-Johnson Temperament Analysis (T-JTA) (Taylor & Morrison, 1984). This scale includes items that indicate personality traits, such as nervousness, impulsiveness, inhibited response, submissiveness, and hostility, which together indicate the person's self-concept, interdependence, and role functioning.

- Social adjustment is the dimension of an individual's well-being that concerns how she or he gets along with other people, how other people react to her or him, and how she or he interacts with social institutions and societal mores. According to RAM, social adjustment indicates the interdependence and role function adaptive modes. Therefore, *social adjustment* is defined as an individual's ability to give and receive love and nurture others, which affects the expectations about how the person functions and relates with others. Social adjustment is measured with a social adjustment scale (Abdel Wahab, 1990) that includes items such as performance at work and in daily life activities, which show the individual's interdependence and role function adaptive modes.

- *Depression* is defined as a common mental disorder that presents with depressed mood, loss of interest or pleasure, feelings of guilt or low self-worth, disturbed sleep or appetite, low energy, and poor concentration. These problems can become chronic or recurrent and lead to substantial impairments in an individual's ability to take care of his or her everyday responsibilities (WHO, 2010). According to RAM, depression indicates the physiologic adaptive mode. Depression is measured using the Beck Depression Inventory (BDI-II) (Beck, Steer, & Brown, 1996), which includes items such sleeping, eating, loss of energy, fatigue, and loss of interest in sex, which together show the individual's physiologic adaptive mode.

In another example, the SolCos model (Soltys and Coats, 1995) in combination with Butler's (1963) life review process and Erickson's (1963) developmental theory was used by (Gaber, 2011) as a theoretical foundation in her doctoral dissertation titled "effect of reminiscence on depression, self-esteem, and life satisfaction among elderly people".

Before 1960, *reminiscence* was seen as a symptom of mental deterioration and actively discouraged in the care of older people (Stinson, and Kirk, 2006). However, Butler's (1963) early work, which described reminiscence as a universal and natural phenomenon for adults of all ages, revolutionized people's attitudes concerning reminiscence. Erikson (1963) espoused the importance of ego integrity, which could be only looking back over one's life and determining that there was meaning or purpose to that life. To avoid despair, one must determine that living was worthwhile and that there was purpose and satisfaction in living.

Butler's theory (1963) extended Erikson's stages (1963) with the belief that ego integrity is attained by recalling one's past from analytical and evaluative perspectives. Butler formulated the concept of the life review, a universal occurrence among older people, which he described as a conscious internal mental process of reviewing one's life. Furthermore, according to Butler, the life review is an adaptive process by which an older person can put his or her life events in proper perspective and work through unresolved conflicts. The life review is carried out through reminiscence, which is retrieval and reporting of past memories.

Building on the theoretical foundation of Erikson (1963) and Butler (1963), Soltys and Coats (1995) developed a framework to help increase the theoretical understanding and utility of reminiscence. This framework includes five stages: antecedent, individual assessment, establishing the therapeutic purposes, choosing a suitable reminiscence therapy modality, and outcome measurements.

Five Stages in the Current Study

The following are the framework's five states.

> *First stage*: Antecedent is initiated because maladjustment has been encountered through the aging process. Therefore, the second stage is initiated.

> *Second stage*: This is the assessment stage that includes the use of standardized psychometric tools or self-reported instruments. This study used the Mini-Mental State Exam (MMSE) scale, Geriatric Depression Scale (GDS), Self-Esteem Scale, UCLA Loneliness Scale, and Life Satisfaction Scale to assess elderly people for depression, cognitive abilities, self-esteem, satisfaction with life, and feeling of loneliness.

> *Third stage*: Therapeutic purposes for the elderly person are established at this stage. Gaber (2011) set a specific goal using the treatment of reminiscence was to examine the effect of this therapeutic intervention on depression, self-esteem, life satisfaction, and loneliness.

Fourth stage: This stage involves choosing a reminiscence modality. This reminiscence should be life reviews, both pleasant and unpleasant, encouraging individual participation in a semi-structured environment.

Final stage: The short-term and long-term effects of this outcome assessment must be considered and evaluated. Gaber (2011) evaluated the effect of the reminiscence in the form of decreasing depression and loneliness and increasing self-esteem and sense of life-satisfaction with the previously mentioned psychometrics and self-reported tool.

Research studies in the maternity and newborn health nursing specialty include doctoral dissertations by Abdel-Monem (2013) and Abu khatwa (2013) in which both researchers used the Neuman systems model (NSM) as the theoretical framework for their studies. Also, in this field, a doctoral dissertation by Elshair (2013) and one by Mohammed (2012) and Omran (2012) in the medical surgical health nursing specialty used Orem self-care theory as the theoretical framework.

NURSING EDUCATION

Nursing theory is an organized and systematic articulation of a set of statements related to questions in the discipline of nursing (Alligood & Tomey, 2002). Theories in education are used to:

- Provide a general focus for curriculum design
- Guide curricular decision making

Theories in nursing in Egypt are taught in these areas:

- Nursing theories are taught only in postgraduate studies in both master's and doctoral courses. For example, the faculty of Nursing-Cairo University are teaching nursing theories in two semesters with 90 hours allocated per semester. The main aim of this course is to provide the students the knowledge and skills to utilize theories in nursing research, education, and practice. Another example is from the faculty of Nursing-Alexandria University where nursing theories are being taught in the doctoral course foundations of nursing science with a total 60 of credit hours. Moreover, nursing theories are being taught in postgraduate courses by the faculty of Nursing-Ain Shams University with a total 45 hours per semester.

USING THEORIES IN NURSING PRACTICE IN EGYPT

One of the most common theories of practice is the nursing process of analyzing assessment data (Croyle, 2005). Theory of nursing process is the most common theory used in nursing practice in Egypt.

Using of nursing process theory in nursing practice in Egypt:

> The nursing process has for many years provided a systematic framework for the delivery of nursing care. Nursing process means the fulfilling of the requirement for a scientific methodology. Nursing process is dynamic, not static. It is an ongoing process that continues for as long as the nurse and client have interactions directed toward change in the client's physical or behavioral responses. The nursing process consists of six steps and uses a problems-solving approach that has come to be accepted as a nursing scientific methodology. It is goal-directed, with the objective of delivering of quality client care.

In Egypt nursing practices are based on the nursing process theory as the nurse provides care for patient/family in the following steps: assessment, analysis, planning, implementation, evaluation, and re-assessment.

CONCLUSION

The use of nursing theories in Egypt is very limited; however, their use for nursing education in Egypt in the future is suggested by the increasing number of students in nursing doctoral programs. The continuous enhancement of the Egyptian nursing education is expected to allow the testing and application of nursing theories in different fields. Many aspects of health care in Egypt need deep and constant nursing research to help nurses provide the best available and suitable nursing care for their patients.

REFERENCES

Abdel Monem, S. A. (2013). *Impact of a structured prenatal counseling on anxiety level among women undergoing intrauterine interventional procedures.* Unpublished doctorate dissertation, Faculty of Nursing, Cairo University.

Abdelsalam, A. Z. (2011). *Effect of supportive psychotherapy on interpersonal problems, personality pathology, and social adjustment among hospitalized depressed women.* Unpublished doctorate dissertation, Faculty of Nursing, Cairo University.

Abdel Wahab, E. (1990). *Measuring social adjustment among schizophrenic patients.* Unpublished doctorate dissertation. Faculty of Nursing, Cairo University.

Abu khatwa, M. A. (2013). *Impact of nutritional protocol of Omega-3 fatty acids on the occurrence of preclampsia among high risk pregnant women: An evidence based approach.* Unpublished doctorate dissertation, Faculty of Nursing, Cairo University.

Alligood, M. R., & Tomey, A. M. (2002). *Nursing theory: Utilization & application* (3rd ed.). St. Louis, Missouri: Elsevier Mosby Publications.

Barkham, M., Hardy, G. E., & Startup, M. (1996). The inventory of problems-32: A short version of the inventory of interpersonal problems. *British Journal of Clinical Psychology*, *35*, 21–35.

Beck, A. T., Steer, R. A., & Brown, G. K. (1996). *Manual for the Beck Depression Inventory—II*. San Antonio, TX: Psychological Corporation.

Butler, R. N. (1963). The life review: An interpretation of reminiscence in the aged. *Psychiatry*, *26*, 65–75.

Crocker, J., & Park, L. E. (2004). *The costly pursuit of self-esteem*. Psychological Bulletin, 130, 392–414.

Crocker, J., & Wolfe, C. T. (2001). *Contingencies of self-worth*. Psychological Review, 108, 593–623.

Croyle, R. T. (2005). *Theory at a glance: Application to health promotion and health behavior* (2nd ed.). Washington, DC: U.S. Department of Health and Human Services, National Institutes of Health. www.thecommunityguide.org

Elshair, A. A. (2013). Mother and child health Al-Quds University: Gestational diabetes in Untied Nation relief and working agency health clinics in Gaza strip: Impact of educational program. Unpublished doctorate dissertation, Faculty of Nursing, Cairo University.

Erickson, E. H. (1963). *Childhood and society* (2nd ed.). New York: Norton.

Fitzpatrick, C. M., & Whall, M. (2005). *Conceptual models of nursing analysis: Synthesis and applications*. Norwalk, CT: B. Lippincott.

Gaber, M. N. (2011). *The effect of reminiscence on depression, self-esteem, and life satisfaction among elderly population*. Unpublished doctorate dissertation, Faculty of Nursing, Cairo University.

George, L., Ellison, C. G., & Larson, D. B. (2002). Explaining the relationships between religious involvement and health. *Journal of Psychological Inquiry*, *13*(3), 190–200.

James, W. (1890). *The principles of psychology*. Cambridge, MA: Harvard University Press.

Kennedy, S., Eisfeld, B., Hons, B., & Cooke, R. (2001). Quality of life: An important dimension in assessing the treatment of depression. *Journal of Psychiatry and Neuroscience*, *26*, 523–528.

Locke, D. (2000). Circumplex Scales of Interpersonal Values: Reliability, validity, and applicability to interpersonal problems and personality disorders. *Journal of Personality Assessment*, *75*, 249–267.

Mohammed, A. H. (2012). *Impact of proposed nursing rehabilitation program on self management of selected side effects of chemotherapy for patients with GIT cancer*. Unpublished doctorate dissertation, Faculty of Nursing, Cairo University.

Omran, S. S. (2012). *Impact of a designed nursing rehabilitation program on patients' outcomes after anterior cruciate ligament (ACL) reconstruction at El-Manial University Hospital*. Unpublished doctorate dissertation, Faculty of Nursing, Cairo University.

Peplau, H. E. (1991). Interpersonal relations in nursing. New York, NY: Springer.

Pargament, K., Koenig, H., Tarakeshwar, N., & Hahn, J. (2004). Religious coping methods as predictors of psychological, physical and spiritual outcomes among medically ill elderly patients: Two-year longitudinal study. *Journal of Health Psychology*, *9*(6), 713–730.

Porter, R., Linsley, K., & Ferrier, N. (2001). Treatment of severe depression-non-pharmacological aspects. *Journal of Advanced Psychiatric Treatment*, *7*, 117–124.

Roy, C., & Andrews, H. A. (1999). The Roy adaptation model (2nd ed.). Stamford, CT: Appleton & Lange.

Roy, C. (1970). Adaptation: A conceptual framework for nursing. *Nursing Outlook*, *18*(3), 42–45.

Soltys, F., & Coats, L. (1995). The SolCos model: Facilitating reminiscence therapy. *Journal of Psychosocial Nursing*, *33*(11), 21–26.

Stinson, C., & Kirk, E. (2006). Structured reminiscence: An intervention to decrease depression and increase self-transcendence in older women. *Journal of Clinical Nursing*, *15*, 208–218.

Taylor, R., & Morrison, L. (1984). *Taylor-Johnson Temperament Analysis Manual*. Los Angeles: Psychological Publications.

World Health Organisation (2010). Mental health and development: Targeting people with mental health conditions as a vulnerable group. WHO Press, Geneva. http://www.who.int/mental_health/policy/development/en/index.html and http://www.psychiatry.uct.ac.za/mhapp/

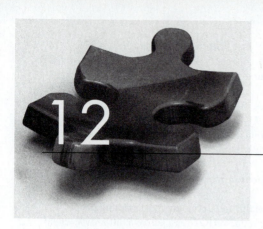

Israel: Applications of Transcultural Nursing Theory

Merav Ben Natan, Mally Ehrenfeld,
and Michal Itzhaki

INTRODUCTION: NURSING IN ISRAEL

Overview of the Israeli Society

Israeli society is culturally diverse, characterized by many different groups of religions and ethnicities (Statistical Abstract of Israel, 2013). Israel is a binational country where Jews and Arabs live side by side. According to the Israel Central Bureau of Statistics (n.d.), Israel's total population had reached 8,134,100 inhabitants by the end of 2013: 75% Jews, 20.7% Arabs, and 4.3% others. The non-Jewish population in Israel is constantly increasing (Ehrenfeld, Itzhaki, & Baumann, 2007).

Of Israel's population, 70.2% was born in Israel, and 29.8% was born elsewhere. Since the establishment of Israel, 3.092 million immigrants have arrived on its shores (Central Bureau of Statistics, 2013). Thus, in Israel, the population is a mixture of cultures that has been altered by an influx of immigrants from various communities including the former Soviet Union, Ethiopia, the United States, and France. The largest of these is the group of immigrants from the former Soviet Union (Ehrenfeld et al., 2007).

Jews have come to Israel during several waves of immigration. Each wave had its own characteristics in terms of geographical origin, causes, dimensions, dominant ideas, and achievements. Israel is unique in its official and long-standing encouragement of Jewish immigration, providing citizenship rights on arrival to the country, accommodation in immigration centers, vocational training, health insurance, welfare, social care, and cash vouchers. This openness to immigration has remained consistent even in times of economic stress and other crises. As a result, Jews have continued to arrive from all over the world to settle in Israel, unlike patterns of immigration and asylum seeking in other countries. These waves of immigration usually include all family members—elderly people, adults, and children, both healthy and sick (Delbar, Tzadok, Mergi, Erel, & Romem, 2010).

The effect of a large number of immigrants on a small society has been highly significant socially, economically, and culturally. The need to absorb newcomers placed a heavy burden on the young state, although once integrated, immigrants contribute considerable economic growth to the country. They bring with them their values and traditions, and these in turn have influenced the emerging society in Israel (Kaplan, 2013).

Different language groups are common in Israel. Hebrew, the language of the Bible, and Arabic are the official languages of the state of Israel (Israeli Ministry of Tourism, 2013). However, many people prefer to speak their own ethnic languages, such as Russian, Amharic, French, Yiddish, English, and Spanish (Noble, Nuszen, Rom, & Noble, 2014). Religion is also diverse: The Arab-speaking population's religion comprises 84.1% Muslims, 8.1% Druze, and 7.8% Arab-Christians. Moreover, religious identity among Israeli Jews is defined differently: secular, orthodox, or ultra-orthodox (Kaplan, 2013).

Within the Jewish Israeli population itself, a complex issue known as the "religious-secular divide" affects Israelis' personal and professional lives and serves as a point of friction in the Israeli Jewish society (Efron, 2003). This divide is a conflict based on geopolitical, theological, and ideological issues. Although the conflict appears to be a polarization of those within the ultra-orthodox and secular Jewish populations, a more inclusive representation also includes the religious and traditional Jewish populations. The four different Jewish religious groups are distinguished one from the other by cultural values, beliefs, and practices (Noble, Engelhardt, Newsome-Wicks, & Woloski-Wruble, 2009).

Israel is also experiencing the increasing phenomenon of foreign workers from all over the world, who come to work in Israel. Therefore, the country has a special web of ethnic groups, customs, languages, beliefs, and values so that cultural diversity is the standard today, and nurses in Israel provide nursing care to patients from diverse cultural backgrounds (Eldar, 2013).

BRIEF DESCRIPTION OF THE ISRAELI HEALTH CARE SYSTEM

The state of Israel was established in 1948. Since that time, government ministries have been organized. In 1949 The Ministry of Health replaced the Mandatory Department of Health and regional health bureaus, and an epidemiological service was formed. The state extended its responsibility for health services by taking over existing hospital facilities inherited from the Mandatory authorities, by building and operating hospitals, and by establishing mother-and-child health care services. The Ministry of Health is responsible for the development of health policy, operation of the nation's public health services, and management of the governmental health care budget. The government also owns and operates many of the nation's large hospitals. It is responsible for licensing those who work in the medical and paramedical professions. In addition, the Ministry initiates and oversees implementation of all health-related legislation passed by the Knesset (Israel Ministry of Foreign Affairs, 2013).

Since the establishment of Israel, the issue of health care has never left the public agenda. The public debate on reform of the health system has focused on the enactment of a national health insurance law. In 1995, The National Health Insurance Law (the official name of this law) went into effect; it stated that participation in a medical insurance plan is compulsory. All Israeli citizens are entitled to basic health care as a fundamental right. Based on this legislation, citizens join one of four health care funds for basic treatment and can increase medical coverage by purchasing supplementary health care (Israel Ministry of Foreign Affairs, 2013). Currently, providers in the Israeli health care system consist of a mixture of private, semiprivate, and public entities (Israeli Medical Association, 2007).

Israel's high standard of health services, modern hospital facilities, and top-quality medical technology and research all contribute to the country's high standard of health today (Israel Ministry of Foreign Affairs, 2013). In a 2013 survey of 48 countries, Israel's health system was ranked fourth in the world in terms of efficiency (Linder-Ganz & Tzach, 2013).

BRIEF DESCRIPTION OF THE NURSING POPULATION IN ISRAEL

Nursing in Israel exists in a unique religious, cultural, historic, and international political context, which provides it a source of identity and ongoing challenges (Ehrenfeld, Itzhaki, & Baumann, 2007). Nurses are the largest group of health care workers in Israel, providing most of its health care (Riba, Greenberger, & Reches, 2004). Nurses in Israel struggle with many of the same problems nurses in other parts of the world face, such as increased use of technology, overwhelming amounts of information, and demands for high quality of services to more people within tighter budgets (Ehrenfeld et al., 2007).

As in other countries, Israel is experiencing a nursing shortage. In 2012, the ratio of employed nurses per 1,000 patients was 5.9, and the ratio of registered nurses per 1,000 patients was 4.8 (Ministry of Health, 2012). Several factors are expected to lead to a greater nursing short- age in Israel including the high rate of population growth, nurses' aging and retirement, increased life expectancy for most people in the country, a dramatic decrease in the number of immigrating nurses, nurses leaving public hospitals for private health care institutions that pay higher salaries and provide better benefits, and leaving the country for higher salaries and better benefits abroad (Ehrenfeld et al., 2007).

In 2012, the nursing workforce in Israel consisted of 82% registered nurses and 18% practical nurses (Ministry of Health, 2012). Nursing edu- cation in the country can be obtained in registered nurse certificate and diploma programs and in academic degree programs offered by universi- ties and colleges (Birenbaum-Carmeli, 2007). Despite the chronic nursing shortage, as part of the professionalization and academization of nursing, the Ministry of Health closed all practical nurse programs. Thus, the pro- portion of registered nurses has grown significantly (Ministry of Health). Moreover, with strong encouragement from the Ministry of Health, the educational programs for registered nurses are being transformed into academic degree programs. In addition to the established university nurs- ing programs, college nursing programs continue to expand (Ehrenfeld et al., 2007).

Increased efficiency and a higher professional level are required of health care workers. Nurses in Israel, as elsewhere, are being given increased responsibilities and are required to have excellent clinical decision-making skills. Advance practice nursing is also increasing, espe- cially in communities and remote locations (Ehrenfeld et al., 2007).

A substantial ethnic diversity exists among Israeli doctors, nurses, and other health care professionals (Delbar, 2006). The composition of the nursing workforce reflects sociodemographic and economic processes in Israel. This workforce comes primarily from two somewhat marginal sub- populations: immigrants from the former Soviet Union and Israeli Arabs (Birenbaum-Carmeli, 2007).

Because of the waves of immigration from the former Soviet Union, Israel received thousands of professionals and highly skilled workers, among them nurses, who have entered the labor market (Khanin, 2010). This changed the nature of the country in general and the health care system in particular. Most immigrant nurses in Israel are from the former Soviet Union (Itzhaki, Ea, Ehrenfeld, & Fitzpatrick, 2013).

Another important source of nurses are immigrants from the former Soviet Union who had previously acquired academic degrees in other fields in their country of origin. These immigrants took advantage of the opportunity to change their previous occupations to nursing through retraining programs offered by the government that sought to reduce the nursing shortage (Khanin, 2010). Physicians and nurses born in the former Soviet Union now constitute 40% of hospital personnel in the Israeli health system (Rassin, 2008).

Another large ethnic group among Israeli nurses is the Arab minority group. The Arab minority in Israel suffers from relatively poor status. This is reflected in lower rates of university-educated professionals and managers versus higher rates of employment in less skilled occupations, such as construction, services (e.g., waiters), and industry work (e.g., factory work). Arabs also suffer from an over-representation in poverty and unemployment rates. Like other minorities, Arabs (both men and women) find the nursing profession to be a bridge toward upward social mobility (Arieli, 2007; Halperin & Mashiach-Eizenberg, 2013).

There is notably a high demand for nursing studies in the group of immigrants from the former Soviet Union, which is also related to sociodemographic and economic processes in Israel. Nursing is perceived as a relatively secure source of livelihood in the country. As such, it is especially attractive in harder times and to people of more modest financial means, such as immigrants (Birenbaum-Carmeli, 2007). This binationality of Israeli nursing emerges as a field of interethnic dialog, thereby modestly contributing to Jewish-Arab coexistence in Israel (Birenbaum-Carmeli, 2007).

USE OF NURSING THEORIES IN ISRAELI NURSING

A *nursing theory* is a set of concepts, definitions, relationships, and assumptions or propositions derived from nursing models or from other disciplines. The theory projects a purposeful, systematic view of phenomena by designing specific inter-relationships among concepts for the purposes of describing, explaining, predicting, and/or prescribing. Nursing theory seeks to describe, predict, and explain the phenomenon of nursing. It provides the foundations of nursing practice, helps to generate further knowledge, and indicates in which direction nursing should develop in the future. Nursing theory can be seen as an attempt by the nursing profession to maintain its professional boundaries (DeKeyser & Medoff-Cooper, 2001).

Israeli nursing is heavily influenced by Western cultures, especially that of the United States, and follows their main trends in nursing research, education, and practice—although this influence is adjusted to the Israeli sociocultural context. Therefore, the use of nursing theories is not new to Israel but have been taught and applied in nursing research and practice. However, the ongoing academization and professionalization processes of Israeli nursing (Spitzer & Perrenoud, 2006), as well as the requirement to follow international high standards, have highlighted the importance of the discussion and use of nursing theories (Ehrenfeld et al., 2007).

USE OF THEORY IN NURSING EDUCATION

Nursing education in Israel is similar to that of other developed countries (Spitzer & Perrenoud, 2006). Among the major theories that are studied in Israeli nursing programs are Leininger's theory of transcultural nursing (theory of culture care: diversity and universality); Orem's self-care theory; Roper, Logan, & Tierney's model of nursing (based upon activities of living); and Watson's theory of human caring. They are studied at the beginning of the programs as part of the course sciences of nursing. Students study the essence of the theory and its contribution to the professional development as a basis for action and research in nursing (Briefings to First Year, 2013). The curriculum is based on Western literature, but as mentioned, it is adjusted to the Israeli sociocultural context.

USE OF THEORY IN NURSING RESEARCH

The core of every research project is its theoretical background, which leads the researcher in planning, performing, and analyzing the researched phenomenon (Eldar, 2013). The development of Israeli nursing research has been followed by a raised awareness and interest in using theories, including nursing theories, as the basis for research. Israeli researchers refine nursing theories and generate nursing knowledge, which is relevant to the Israeli sociocultural context (DeKeyser & Medoff-Cooper, 2001).

USE OF THEORY IN NURSING PRACTICE

The main problem is the gap between the nursing theories that are taught in Israeli nursing programs and the practice of Israeli nurses; this is also frequently encountered in other countries. One reason for this gap is the difficulty of translating theory into practice (DeKeyser & Medoff-Cooper,

2001). Numerous Israeli studies based on nursing theories provide recommendations for improving nursing practice. However, their implementation is slow. Another reason for the theory-practice gap is nurses' resistance to change well-established routines. Fear of the unknown and distrust of new ideas also play a part in slowing the process of theory implementation (Eldar, 2013).

TRANSCULTURAL NURSING IN ISRAELI NURSING RESEARCH, EDUCATION, AND PRACTICE

Nurses in Israel come from diverse cultural backgrounds and care for patients of diverse cultural backgrounds. Cultural and ethnic diversity in Israeli society can influence the interaction between health care providers and their patients. This can be frustrating for both sides and is often blamed on cultural differences and difficulties in communication (Delbar, 2006). Evidence indicates that health care, which is culturally, religiously, and linguistically adequate, improves compliance to treatment and the treatment's outcomes (Eldar, 2013).

Each individual, family, and community can have cultural and behavioral characteristics that influence health and illness situations and require specific cultural attitudes. This requires caregivers to learn about different cultures and to explore and understand the most suitable methods for helping patients according to their unique needs (Leininger, 1991; Leininger & McFarland, 2002).

Realizing that care and culture are inextricably linked and cannot be separated in nursing care actions and decisions Leininger (1988) launched her theory of culture care: diversity and universality (CCDU) with the goal of providing culturally congruent, holistic care. Culturally congruent care means providing care measures that are in harmony with the cultural beliefs, practices, and values of an individual or group (Sitzman & Eichelberger, 2011). The central purposes of this theory are to discover and explain diverse and universal, culturally based care factors that influence the health, well-being, illness, or death of individuals or groups and to use research findings to provide culturally congruent, safe, and meaningful care to patients of diverse or similar cultures (Leininger, 2002).

Leininger's theory is the primary, comprehensive transcultural nursing theory used in Israel today. Leininger developed its concepts in the mid-1950s. Transcultural nursing is a humanistic and scientific area of formal study and practice in nursing that focuses on differences and similarities among cultures with respect to human care, health, and illness based on people's cultural values, beliefs, and practices (Leininger, 1991).

Leininger's (1991) sunrise model is a part of CCDU. It describes the various dimensions of culture that are meaningful in explaining health and well-being. According to the model, nursing care bridges generic or folk systems and professional systems—two major constructs of the CCDU theory (Sagar, 2012).

Another model of transcultural nursing is the model for developing cultural competence by Papadopoulos, Tilki, and Taylor (1998). *Competence* is the ability to use knowledge and skills in professional and personal development. It can also be described in terms of responsibility and autonomy (The European Qualifications Framework, 2008). When relating to nursing and other health professionals, *cultural competence* is the ability to provide effective health care, considering the patient's beliefs, behaviors, habits, and needs, according to their cultural background (Papadopoulos, 2006).

The model for developing cultural competence by Papadopoulos, Tilki, and Taylor (1998) is composed of four stages: cultural awareness, cultural knowledge, cultural sensitivity, and cultural competence. Cultural competence is a process as well as an output and requires the combining of knowledge and skills that are constantly acquired during a person's personal and professional lives (Papadopoulos, 2008).

Concepts of transcultural nursing are especially relevant to countries characterized by cultural diversity, such as Israel. Therefore, the present work focuses on the role of transcultural nursing and the use of its theories and models in Israeli nursing research, education, and practice.

NURSING RESEARCH

The cultural and ethnic diversity of the Israeli society and the growing awareness of the importance of the culture dimension in providing patients with appropriate care (Eldar, 2013) have led to many nursing studies in Israel based on the theoretical concepts of transcultural nursing and the exploration of a variety of populations and health care fields. Israeli researchers used these studies to generate knowledge related to cultural care. Some of the studies focus on patients whereas others focus on nurse populations. Some focus on the dimension of culture in provision and reception of nursing care and others on various subjects relevant to nurse population.

For example, Delbar et al. (2010) found that sociocultural differences between immigrants and the host society and the lack of awareness of these differences by mental health professionals might influence rates and patterns of psychiatric hospitalization. Another example is the work of Sheiner, Sheiner, Hershkovitz, Mazor, Katz, and Shoham-Vardi (2000), which investigated factors affecting the ability of obstetricians and midwives to estimate the pain intensity level of low-risk women in early active labor. Both the caretakers and patients were asked to assess the patients' labor pain. Results revealed that the staff appropriately assessed the intensity level of pain correctly in only half of the entire sample. The discrepancy was significantly correlated with religiosity and parity. The pain intensity levels of most secular patients were assessed correctly, but that of a significant number of the religious parturients were underestimated, especially the pain of most of the grand multiparous women. With a mostly secular staff, the researchers hypothesized that the inaccuracies in level of pain intensity might have been influenced by the cultural gap between the staff and the patients. However, it is important to note that ethnic attitudes of the staff were not measured in the reported study; therefore, the hypothesis could not be confirmed.

Research has consistently demonstrated that health care providers should make every effort to familiarize themselves with the cultural backgrounds and identities of their patients and become competent to engage actively and in the spirit of partnership with their patients in order to provide them appropriate and acceptable care (Delbar et al., 2010; Noble et al., 2009).

Many researchers realize that culture dimension is relevant to the nurse population itself because nurses function in a sociocultural context, and their cultural norms and values might shape their attitudes toward various topics (Rassin, 2008). For example, Arieli (2007) explored the implications for Arab enrolled nurses in Israel facing the academization of nursing. She found that the women's negative attitudes to the conversion course were not related to their otherwise positive attitudes to education in general. The conversion course was affected by adverse material conditions, cultural factors, and feelings of helplessness. The threat of the loss of their professional nursing status as a result of the changes in nursing gave rise to a great sense of personal loss. The researcher concluded that as reported in other countries, the academization of nursing in Israel is obstructing one of the major routes of social mobility for women in the weaker sections of society. This situation is experienced as particularly harsh because of the overall oppressive situation that Arab women in Israel suffer.

Another subject for research is the integration of immigrant nurses into a host culture. The process by which immigrant nurses integrate into a host culture is complex and multidimensional (Ea, Itzhaki, Ehrenfeld, & Fitzpatrick, 2010). Nursing studies that investigate acculturation among immigrant nurses lend support to the concepts of acculturation theorized by Leininger (1995). For example, Ea et al. explored the levels of acculturation of the large group of nurses in Israel from the Soviet Union. Their study results indicate that this group has a stronger affinity to their original culture than the Israeli culture. The major factor that could have contributed to this group's level of acculturation is the strong presence and continued influence of the Russian culture in Israel. As a result, there may be limited opportunities for sustained and constant exposure to the norms and behaviors of the host culture.

NURSING EDUCATION

Training nurses to provide transcultural nursing is important in order to assist them in increasing their sensitivity to culturally diverse communities and to care for patients from different cultures with respect and dignity. Cultural diversity was determined as a topic that should be included in the core curriculum by the Israeli Ministry of Health (2005). Currently, transcultural nursing and its theories and models are studied as part of the basic nursing program, but specific requirements for a course in transcultural nursing have not been delineated (Noble et al., 2014). At times, transcultural nursing was not a part of the compulsory curriculum of nursing schools and nursing departments. This means that most nurses in Israel practice nursing care that is not based on formal transcultural education (Eldar, 2013).

According to Yellon's (2012) and Eldar's (2013) studies, nurses assert that there is a lack of training in cultural competence in Israel. It should be noted that some studies have demonstrated that nurses show great interest and motivation in gaining knowledge and skills in transcultural nursing (Eldar, 2013; Yellon, 2012). Indeed, the Israeli Ministry of Health began a process for cultural and linguistic compatibility and access in the health system as was published in a management circular whose instructions were implemented in February 2013. The circular emphasized that to cope with cultural diversities and the variety of languages, human values as well as legal aspects must be considered when defining reasonable and proper medical service. In other words, a standard of care must be determined. The circular instructed health organizations to prepare an outline for cultural and linguistic compatibility and access and to train one member of the management staff of each health organization (hospital or clinics) to be a cultural competence coordinator who would implement the cultural standards in the organization. It also recommended that all the health services staff participate in cultural competence courses (Eldar, 2013).

In Israel, nursing students are culturally diverse. Teaching a diverse student body can be difficult. It requires avoiding unwanted discrimination and treating everyone in the same way regardless of race, ethnicity, country of origin, gender, age, socioeconomic status, or any other characteristic. Moreover, there is a need to develop strategies for working with nontraditional students (Bednarz, Schim, & Doorenbos, 2010).

According to Leininger, nurses need to understand the patients' worlds, to learn from their backgrounds, and to explore the culturally appropriate ways for helping them to become and stay healthy (Leininger, 1991; Leininger & McFarland, 2002). Such an approach has been applied by Israeli nurse educators in teaching a diverse student body; this involves showing respect and tolerance to each one's cultural diversity and helping students succeed in accordance with each one's cultural norms and values (Rassin, 2008).

An example of learning about diverse students' backgrounds is Israeli nursing schools' tradition of organizing ethnic potluck lunches at the beginning of the nursing program. Teachers and students can sample the deliciously strange foods of other cultures and see people wearing traditional outfits. This often is followed by a panel discussion about what various groups need and want.

NURSING PRACTICE

To provide culturally congruent nursing, nurses in Israel are required to develop cultural competence toward patients' cultural needs with transcultural care decisions and actions (Noble et al., 2014). But are Israeli nurses indeed culturally competent? Several studies based on the model for developing cultural competence (Papadopoulos, Tilki, & Taylor, 1998) that explored cultural competence among the Israeli nurses have demonstrated that nurses lack knowledge of it. Consequently, these nurses lack confidence in providing nursing care to patients of diverse cultural backgrounds (Eldar, 2013; Yellon, 2012). In contrast, Noble's (2005) study of the cultural competence and ethnic attitudes of 30 Israeli midwives from a major hospital in Jerusalem concerning Orthodox Jewish couples in labor and delivery found that midwives were culturally aware, culturally competent, and culturally proficient.

In Eldar's (2013) study, cultural competence was perceived to be higher among nurses who often provided care for patients of various cultural backgrounds. The non-Jewish nurses were perceived to be more culturally competent. Cultural competence also largely depends on preparedness by training courses.

Nissim (2010) explored the experience of six nurses originally from Ethiopia who were providing care to patients from different cultural backgrounds in Israel. The findings revealed that the experience of caring for patients from a culture different from the one of the nurses is an exhausting cognitive activity, involving constant attentiveness. The nurses were highly aware that some of their nursing care behaviors originated from their cultural heritage and were able to distinguish between personal cultural values and generic cultural features. This self-awareness apparently forms the basis for the nurses' ability to develop skills of cultural competence.

Leininger (2006) has proposed three action modes for providing culturally congruent, holistic nursing care in health and well-being or when dealing with illness or dying: preservation and/or maintenance, accommodation and/or negotiation, and repatterning and/or restructuring. *Preservation and/or maintenance* refers to those decisions that maintain and preserve desirable and helpful values and beliefs. *Accommodation and/or negotiation* is helpful in the adaptation and transaction for care that is fitting for the culture of the individual, families, or groups. *Repatterning and/or restructuring* involve mutual decision-making process as the nurse modifies or changes the nursing action to achieve better health outcomes.

Israeli nurses often naturally practice these action modes. For example, accommodation and/or negotiation between the generic care and the professional care-cure practices in Israeli health care is expressed through the involvement of rabbis in health and illness decisions of Orthodox or Ultra-Orthodox Jews, such as the Hassidic Jews (Coleman-Brueckheimer & Dein, 2011; Ivry, 2010). The spiritual leader of Hassidic Jews is a rabbi, so by consulting with one regarding their health and illness conditions, patients seek to ensure that their actions are in accord with God's will and that they fulfill their responsibilities as believing Ultra-Orthodox Jews (Coleman-Brueckheimer & Dein). This example represents cultural norm and practice that is known and accepted by the majority of the Israeli society.

RECRUITMENT OF NURSES

Ethnically diverse health care providers are needed to ensure a high quality of health care delivery in Israel. Another important subject indirectly related to nursing practice is the role of the cultural dimension in the recruitment of nurses. A workforce of culturally diverse registered nurses strengthens the delivery of culturally competent care and is better equipped than a primarily singular cultural care to contribute to positive minority (non-Jewish) patient outcomes and to patient satisfaction. Moreover, there is evidence that patients prefer health care providers who share their racial or ethnic background (Sullivan Commission, 2004).

The efforts of Israeli stakeholders to recruit nurses to expand the diversity among registered nurses in the labor market (Arieli & Hirschfeld, 2013) prove their awareness of the importance of the culture dimension in nursing care (Ben Natan & Oren, 2011). Efforts to expand the diversity among registered nurses have included a variety of strategies, such as training second career professionals, increasing financial compensation for nurses in the workforce, and improving workplace conditions (Ben Natan & Oren, 2011).

SUMMARY

This chapter provides an overview of the use of nursing theories in Israeli nursing research, education, and practice and in the country's sociocultural context while focusing on the concepts of transcultural nursing and its theories and models. Israel is a culturally diverse country; therefore, transcultural nursing is especially relevant to discuss in the Israeli context. The chapter presented various examples of applying the concepts of transcultural nursing and its theories and models in Israeli nursing research, education, and practice. There is rising awareness and interest in using nursing theories in general, although—as has been noted—there are also certain problems in applying those theories, resulting in a theory-practice gap. The ongoing processes of professionalization and academization of Israeli nursing are expected to lift the profile of theories in nursing. The processes are slow and not without pitfalls, but it seems that Israeli nursing is on the right track.

REFERENCES

Arieli, D. (2007). Academization of nursing in Israel: implications for Arab-Israeli nurses. *International Nursing Review, 54*(1), 70–77.

Arieli, D., & Hirschfeld, M. (2013). Supporting minority nursing students: 'Opportunity for success' for Ethiopian immigrants in Israel. *International Nursing Review, 60*(2), 213–220.

Bednarz, H., Schim, S., & Doorenbos, A. (2010). Cultural diversity in nursing education: Perils, pitfalls, and pearls. *Journal of Nursing Education, 49*(5), 253–260.

Ben Natan, M., & Oren, M. (2011). The essence of nursing in the shifting reality of Israel today. *Online Journal of Issues in Nursing, 16*. doi: 10.3912/OJIN.Vol16No02PPT04

Birenbaum-Carmeli, D. (2007). Contextualizing nurse education in Israel: Sociodemography, labor market dynamics and professional training. *Contemporary Nurse, 24*(2), 117–127.

Briefings to First Year. (2013). *Briefings to First Year, 2013–2014*. Tel-Aviv: University of Tel-Aviv, Faculty of Medicine, School of Health Professions.

Central Bureau of Statistics. (2013). *Report on the demographic situation in Israel, 2011*. Retrieved from http://www.cbs.gov.il/reader/?MIval=cw_usr_view_SHTML&ID=629

Coleman-Brueckheimer, K., & Dein, S. (2011). Health care behaviours and beliefs in Hassidic Jewish populations: A systematic review of the literature. *Journal of Religious and Health, 50*, 422–436.

DeKeyser, F., & Medoff-Cooper, B. (2001). A non-theorist's perspective on nursing theory: Issues of the 1990s. *Scholarly Inquiry for Nursing Practice, 15*(4), 329–341.

Delbar, V. (2006). Transcultural health care in Israel: Past history and current issues, In I. Papadopoulos (Ed.), *Transcultural health and social care: The development of culturally competent practitioners*. Edinburgh: Churchill Livingstone Elsevier, 283–301.

Delbar, V., Tzadok, L., Mergi, O., Erel, T. O., Haim, L., & Romem, P. (2010). Transcultural mental health care issues of Ethiopian immigration to Israel. *Advances in Mental Health, 9*(3), 277–287.

Ea, E., Itzhaki, M., Ehrenfeld, M., & Fitzpatrick, J. (2010). Acculturation among immigrant nurses in Israel and the United States of America. *International Nursing Review, 57*(4), 443–448.

Efron, N. J. (2003). *Real Jews: Secular vs. ultra-orthodox and the struggle for Jewish identity in Israel*. New York: Basic Books.

Ehrenfeld, M., Itzhaki, M., & Baumann, S. (2007). Nursing in Israel. *Nursing Science Quarterly, 20*(4), 372–375.

Eldar, O. (2013). *Cultural competence among hospital nurses in Israel*. Unpublished doctoral dissertation, Babeş-Bolyai University. Retrieved from http://www.google.co.il/url?sa=t&rct=j&q=&esrc=s&source=web&cd=2&ved=0CCMQFjAB&url=http%3A%2F%2F193.231.20.119%2Fdoctorat%2Fteza%2Ffisier%2F1756&ei=cdHWVJPfHMPxavLIgKgB&usg=AFQjCNGJMUcNqFOAWGYc-p3JuBdmkuyBLg&bvm=bv.85464276,d.d2s

European Qualifications Framework. (2008). *Recommendation of the European Parliament and of the Council*. Retrieved from from http://eurlex.europa.*eu*/LexUriServ/LexUriServ.do?uri=OJ:C:*2008*:111:0001

Halperin, O., & Mashiach-Eizenberg, M. (2013). Becoming a nurse—A study of career choice and professional adaptation among Israeli Jewish and Arab nursing students: A quantitative research study. *Nurse Education Today*. doi: 10.1016/j.nedt.2013.10.001

Israel Central Bureau of Statistics. (n.d.). *Population, by population group*. Retrieved from http://www1.cbs.gov.il/publications13/yarhon0413/pdf/b1.pdf

Israeli Medical Association. (2007). *Sherutei refuah pratit (Sharap)—2007* [Private sector healthcare services—2007]. Retrieved from http://www.ima.org.il/mainsite/ViewCategory.aspx?CategoryId=930

Israel Ministry of Foreign Affairs. (2013). *The healthcare system in Israel—An historical perspective*. Retrieved from http://mfa.gov.il/MFA/AboutIsrael/IsraelAt50/Pages/The%20Health%20Care%20System%20in%20Israel-%20An%20Historical%20Pe.aspx

Israeli Ministry of Health. (2005). *Mandated course curriculum for registered nurses—2006*. Jerusalem: Author.

Israeli Ministry of Tourism. (2013). *Languages in Israel*. Retrieved from http://www.goisrael.com/Tourism_Eng/Tourist%20Information/Discover%20Israel/Pages/Languages.aspx

Itzhaki, M., Ea, E., Ehrenfeld, M., & Fitzpatrick, J. (2013). Job satisfaction among immigrant nurses in Israel and in the United States of America. *International Nursing Review, 60*, 122–128. doi: j.1466-7657.2012.01035.x

Ivry, T. (2010). Kosher medicine and medicalized halacha: An exploration of triadic relations among Israeli rabbis, doctors and infertility patients. *American Ethnologist, 37*(4), 662–680.

Kaplan, J. (2013). *Introduction: The diversity of Israeli society*. Jerusalem:The Jewish Agency for Israel. Retrieved from http://jafi.org/JewishAgency/English/Jewish+Education/Compelling+Content/Eye+on+Israel/Society/1)+Introduction+The+Diversity+of+Israeli+Society.htm

Khanin, V. (2010). *Aliyah from the former Soviet Union: Contribution to the national security balance*. Position paper presented to the 10th Annual Herzliya Conference, Herzliya, Israel, on the behalf of the Israeli Ministry of Immigrant Absorptions.

Leininger, M. M. (1988). Leininger's theory of nursing: Cultural care diversity and universality. *Nursing Science Quarterly, 1*(4), 152–160.

Leininger, M. M. (1991). *Culture care diversity & universality: A theory of nursing.* New York: National League for Nursing Press.

Leininger, M. (1995). *Transcultural nursing: Concepts, theories, research and practices* (2nd ed.). New York: McGraw-Hill.

Leininger, M. (2002). Culture care theory: A major contribution to advance transcultural nursing knowledge and practices. *Journal of Transcultural Nursing, 13*(3), 189–192.

Leininger, M. M. (2006). Culture care diversity and universality and evolution of the ethnonursing method. In M. Leininger & M. McFarland (Eds.), *Culture care diversity and universality: A worldwide nursing theory* (pp. 1–41). Sudbury, MA: Jones and Bartlett.

Leininger, M. M., & McFarland, M. R. (2002). *Transcultural nursing. Concepts, theories, research & practice* (3rd ed.). New York: McGraw-Hill.

Linder-Ganz, R., & Tzach, R. (2013, August 28). Israel's healthcare system ranked fourth in world; U.S. trails behind. *Haaretz.* Retrieved from http://www.haaretz.com/news/national/.premium-1.544034

Ministry of Health. (2012). *Duah 2012, Yaadey 2013* [The 2012 report, the goals of 2013]. Jerusalem: Ministry of Health, Nursing Division.

Nissim, S. (2010). *Culturally diverse nurses and the meaning of cultural competence: Ethiopian origin nurses' experiences, caring for culturally different patients.* Germany: VDM Verlag Dr. Müller.

Noble, A., Engelhardt, K., Newsome-Wicks, M., & Woloski-Wruble, A. (2005). Cultural competence and ethnic attitudes of Israeli midwives concerning Orthodox Jewish couples in labor and delivery. *Journal of Midwifery & Women's Health, 50*(5), 441–441.

Noble, A., Engelhardt, K., Newsome-Wicks, M., & Woloski-Wruble, A. C. (2009). Cultural competence and ethnic attitudes of midwives concerning Jewish couples. *Journal of Obstetric, Gynecologic, & Neonatal Nursing, 38*(5), 544–555.

Noble, A., Nuszen, E., Rom, M., & Noble, L. M. (2014). The effect of cultural competence educational intervention for first-year student in Israel. *Journal of Transcultural Nursing, 25*(1), 87–94.

Papadopoulos, I. (2006). *Transcultural health and social care: Development of culturally competent practitioners.* Edinburgh: Churchill Livingstone Elsevier.

Papadopoulos, I. (2008). *The Papadopoulos, Tilki and Taylor model for developing cultural competence.* http://www.ieneproject.eu/download/Outputs/intercultural%20model.pdf

Papadopoulos, I., Tilki, M., & Taylor, G. (1998). *Transcultural care: A guide for health care professionals.* Dinton: Quay Books.

Rassin, M. (2008). Nurses' professional and personal values. *Nursing Ethics, 15*(5), 614–630.

Riba, S., Greenberger, C., & Reches, H. (2004). State involvement in professional nursing development in Israel: Promotive or restrictive. *Online Journal of Issues in Nursing, 9*(3), 10.

Sagar, P. L. (2012). *Transcultural nursing theory and models. Application in nursing education, practice, and administration.* New York: Springer.

Sheiner, E., Sheiner, E., Hershkovitz, R., Mazor, M., Katz, M., & Shoham-Vardi, I. (2000). Overestimation and underestimation of labor pain. *European Journal of Obstetrics & Gynecology and Reproductive Biology, 91*(1), 37–40.

Sitzman, K., & Eichelberger, L. W. (2011). *Understanding the work of nurse theorists: A creative beginning* (2nd ed.). Sudbury, MA: Jones and Bartlett.

Spitzer, A., & Perrenoud, B. (2006). Reforms in nursing education across Western Europe: From agenda to practice. *Journal of Professional Nursing, 22*(3), 150–161.

Statistical Abstract of Israel. (2013). *Selected data from the Statistical Abstract of Israel 2013-No.64*. Retrieved from http://www.cbs.gov.il/reader/shnatonenew_site.htm

Sullivan Commission (2004). *Missing persons: Minorities in the health professions. A report of the Sullivan Commission on Diversity in the Healthcare Workforce*. Available at http://www.healthdiversity.pitt.edu/about/documents/SullivanTaskForceJune_26_FINAL_REPORT_000.pdf

Yellon, T. (2012). *Cultural competence of Israeli nurses*. Unpublished master's thesis, Tel Aviv: Open University, Israel.

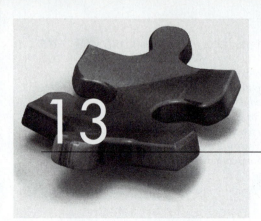

Jordan: Nursing in the Arab World: An Aspiration for a Culturally-Sensitive Nursing Model

Muayyad M. Ahmad and Latefa A. Dardas

INTRODUCTION

In Arab Muslim communities, health beliefs, practices, and education are linked to spiritual and cultural values (AbuGharbieh & Suliman, 1992; Al-Darazi, 2003). Theories from the Western nursing perspective might not be congruent with the beliefs of an Arab Muslim community. Over the past 50 years, the transcultural nursing model has been established as a formal area of inquiry and practice to transform nursing and provide culturally congruent and responsible care to people from diverse cultures (Leininger, 1995). However, no serious attempt has been made yet in the Arab world to build a formal nursing model that resembles what has been developed in Western societies.

Western nursing models developed over the past seven centuries are difficult to apply in the Arab world. Thus, the question is whether *is it better to have a global nursing model that fits cross-culturally, or to create a model tailored to each specific culture?* The Western nursing models with unicultural scope have not contributed significantly to move Arab Muslim's nurses into a global transcultural nursing world. People are looking for care that is culturally congruent, meaningful, and personally helpful to them and their families.

Recently, researchers have recognized the need for a more holistic view of health that integrates Middle-Eastern culture and philosophical concepts into Western approaches for health care. Among the important aspects that need to be considered when developing a model for Arabs are the embrace of Islamic health beliefs, the role of the family, the poor perception of nursing in the community, and the distinct gender roles (Emami, Benner, & Ekman, 2001). However, reaching this target of holistic approaches to health care remains challenging for Arab Muslims because the health belief system in this culture presents spiritual wellness as a prerequisite for the health of body and mind (Wehbe-Alamah, 2008). Thus, a model (or models) of nursing care based on Islamic beliefs is needed to ensure congruence between the Arab culture, Islamic identity, and the practice of nursing care.

ARAB CULTURE: AN OVERVIEW

Arabs are defined by their genealogical, linguistic, and cultural grounds, and not by race. They inhabit Western Asia, North Africa, and parts of the Horn of Africa. There are 22 Arab countries that are religiously and ethnically homogenous with Islam being the dominant religion in most of them. The total number of Arabs living in Arab nations is approximately 366 million. The total number living in non-Arab states is about 17 million. The worldwide total number of Arabs is about 383 million. Only approximately 20% of Muslims around the world are Arabs. The world's largest Muslim community is in Indonesia, which is a non-Arab country. On the other hand, more than 90% of Arabs are Muslims. The Arab homeland covers an area of 5.25 million square miles. By comparison, the United States comprises 3.6 million square miles. With 72% of its territory in Africa and 28% in Asia, the Arab world straddles two continents, a position that makes it one of the world's most strategic regions. Ethnic Arab peoples have one of the world's highest rates of population growth and constitute a significant and increasing population in countries as Australia, Canada, France, Britain, and the United States. Jordan is a small developing Arab country with limited natural resources located in the Middle East. Its estimated population reached 6.5 million by the end of 2012 (Jordan Department of Statistics [DOS], 2013).

Arabs culture is defined by its essential twin constituents of Arabism and Islam. Arab culture is a term that draws together the common themes and overtones found in the Arab countries, especially those of the Middle Eastern countries. Arabs have a shared set of traditions, belief systems, and behaviors shaped by their distinct history, religion, ethnic identity, language, and nationality (Nydell, 2005). Furthermore, although vast social differences exist across different Arab countries, Arabs are more homogenous than Westerners in their outlook on life. Most Arabs share basic beliefs and values that cross national and social class boundaries. Child-rearing practices are nearly identical, and the family structure is essentially the same with a high regard for tradition. Ethnic identity remains important for Arabs, regardless of whether they share the same religion. Their cultural background, education, and native city and country are also important to them. Similarly, their dignity, honor, and reputation are important, and they spare no effort to protect them. Overall, Arabs are united in a shared culture that is considered substantially different from their Western counterparts (Retso, 2002). However, one main characteristic of the Arab culture is its acceptance of the contributions of other races, peoples, and followers of other religions and faiths that coexisted within the Arab-Islamic society.

In Arab culture, the family rather than the individual is the core of the community. The family unit in Islam emerges from a legal marriage. Both males and females are expected to abstain from behaviors that are forbidden by Islam, such as having pre- or extramarital sex (Al-Khayat, 1997). Family relationship is built on respect and privacy. Extended family is also a common phenomenon in the Arab culture, and it entails providing possible economic benefits and helping in children's rearing and elderly care giving. A good relationship between the mother and the child can uphold harmony in the child's behavior and prevent adverse effects of stressors on the mother and distress on child behavior. Young individuals are socialized to respect their elders, be loyal to their family, and to obey their parents (Dhami & Sheikh, 2008). Elderly parents are valued and respected for their life experiences, wisdom, and hierarchical position within the family. Recognition of such diversities among cultures is necessary to design and conduct valid and reliable research as well as accurate cross-cultural programs. Indeed, when Western culture is often offered as the ultimate choice for all peoples, regardless of their heritage or culture, a culturally sensitive approach is considered important to promote pluralism within globalization.

NURSING AS A PROFESSION IN THE ARAB COUNTRIES

Historically, nursing has not been regarded as a prestigious occupation in many Arab countries, and it continues to be regarded with notable reservation. To address this issue, nurses in Saudi Arabia, an Arab country with strong attachment to Islam, benefited from their religion and history to place the nursing profession within a religious framework, which had a positive effect on the perception of nursing as a profession for women (Lovering, 2008). In Arab history, nursing care in the Middle East precedes the era of Florence Nightingale. The first Muslim nurse was Rufaidah Al-Asalmiya, who lived in the eighth century during the time of the Prophet Muhammad (peace be upon him) (Bryant, 2003; Jan, 1996). Recognizing Rufaidah as the first Muslim nurse is a recent phenomenon.

People view nursing in the Middle East as having a low status and compromised moral standing (El-Sanabary, 1993; Harper, 2006). Low status results from many possible factors such as misperception of nurses' roles, consideration of the work as degrading, confusion regarding multiple levels of entry into practice, and the domination of the medical profession over nursing (Al-Aitah, Cameron, Armstrong-Stassen, & Horsburgh, 1999). Barriers to nursing study in the Arab countries could also include the social image of a working female, long working hours over weekends and nights, and low salaries. This image in the society has been reflected in the nursing programs in many Arab countries by the low enrollment of students. Conversely, in the last 15 years, a dramatic change in enrollment to study nursing occurred in Jordan. Currently, 16 nursing schools offer bachelor's degrees in nursing, 4 schools offer master's degrees in different nursing specialties, and 1 school offers a doctor of philosophy degree. Furthermore, the percentage of male nursing students enrolled in nursing programs has reached 65% in the past few years, which potentially reflects a positive change in Jordanian society's perception of the nursing profession. In the past five years, Jordan has witnessed no shortage in nursing staff, and the unemployment figures in nursing have been high.

NURSING EDUCATION SYSTEM IN JORDAN

There are four levels of education to prepare nurses in the Arab countries: high school certification, diploma (two years after high school), associate degree (three years after high school), and bachelor degree (four years after high school). There are few master's degree programs in Jordan, Lebanon, and Egypt, and only two doctoral programs in Egypt and Jordan.

In Jordan, the goal of nursing schools is to assist students to develop skills of critical thinking, problem solving, knowledge synthesis, and nursing behavior that are responsive to present and emerging health care needs. The philosophies of nursing schools in Jordan are congruent with the country's health, social, and economic priorities, which are to improve the education and develop leadership potential in nursing to be able to provide high-quality, safe, and competent health care for all Jordanians and non-Jordanians. Faculty members in these schools believe that professional nursing practice is dynamic, complex, and integral to the health care system. Professional nursing practice adheres to an established framework of ethical principles, legal nursing regulations, and standards of practice.

Arab nurses have expressed concerns that their current nursing education stems from Western philosophy, which is not always consistent with their cultural and religious beliefs or those of Muslim communities (Lovering, 2008; Rassool, 2004). In Jordan, as in other Arab countries, nursing curricula were founded on Western nursing models. Most of the resources for nursing education are not written in the national Arabic language and do not reflect a culturally competent practice. Cultural competence is abstractly presented through the nursing theory course, which is an introductory class at the master's level and an advance course in the Ph.D. program. Separating cultural competence from courses that develop practice skills have made it difficult to relate to practice. Therefore, integrating cultural competence into existing courses is required so that students have an opportunity to see its implications and apply its principles in a variety of contexts. Indeed, concerns have been raised in the past two decades about the influence of the U.S. philosophy of nursing on universities' curricula in Jordan and have suggested that nurses must decide whether the U.S. version of nursing fits Jordanian culture and society (AbuGharbieh & Suliman, 1992).

NURSING MODELS AND ARABS

The purpose of understanding each patient's religion and belief includes the idea that all basic human needs are the same but that culture influences the way those needs are met. Many theories have tried to examine the meaning of caring in the Arab Muslim community. Arab scholars have an increased awareness of the need of a nursing model based on Arab cultural values that can suit Muslim nurses and Arab communities (Lovering, 2008; Rassool, 2004). As a result, research focusing on the nursing values and beliefs practiced within the Arab culture has recently started to appear.

Western-derived models of care influence nursing education and practice in the Middle East because no other model of nursing is available and the number of nursing textbooks written in Arabic is limited (Al-Darazi, 2003). Therefore, nursing programs in Arab countries use a Western-based nursing curriculum. Making models that are congruent with the cultural and religious beliefs of Arab Muslim nurses and their patients has many challenges.

The health beliefs and practices of Arab Muslims are derived from spiritual and cultural values. The need for identifying culturally distinct aspects of caring for Arab Muslim patients in the Middle East has become clear. A large number of non-Muslim nurses, predominantly from India and the Philippines, work in Arab countries. It would be beneficial for these nurses to develop an understanding that their professional belief systems must be adjusted in order to provide care that is harmonious with the beliefs and culture of their patients. The following are a few nursing models that attempt to adjust the Western models to respond to Arab and Muslim societies.

Crescent Model

A thoughtful attempt for meeting the holistic needs of Arab Muslim patients was made through the development of the Crescent of Care nursing model. Cultural, spiritual, and professional nursing values are used to define patients' spiritual, cultural, psychosocial, interpersonal, and clinical caring needs (Lovering, 2008). The main goal of nursing care is to restore the patient's health. In the center of the model are the patient and family as the focus of care, reflecting the cultural importance of family as the primary social unit in Arab culture.

The Crescent model of nursing care illustrates the ethics and beliefs that impact the care of Arab Muslim patients and the units of caring action. This model comes from an ethnographic study of the health beliefs and care meanings of Arab Muslim nurses caring for Arab Muslim patients in the Middle East region. However, a researcher who was not born into the Arab culture developed this model in Saudi Arabia and primarily fits the Saudi culture but not that of other Arab populations.

Leininger Transcultural Model

Transcultural nursing was developed because of the need to work with people from widely divergent cultural atmospheres. Leininger and McFarland (2002) defined transcultural nursing as "a learned, humanistic and scientific profession/discipline that focuses on human care and caring activities to assist, support or facilitate individuals or groups to maintain/regain their health/wellbeing" (p.46). Furthermore, Leininger stated that nursing is essentially a transcultural phenomenon and that knowledge about patients' cultural values, beliefs, and practices is integral to providing holistic nursing care.

Leininger's theory of transcultural care was used to study Arab Muslim immigrant culture care meaning in the United States and in Australia (Wehbe-Alamah, 2005). However, many theorists argue that the meaning of care within one culture will not be the same as when it is in a different culture.

The context of nursing in Jordan draws on the interrelated aspects of Islam, Islamic health beliefs, the importance of family as the primary social unit, and distinct gender roles. Jordan is largely dominated by Muslims (95%, Christians 5%); thus, Leininger's theory applies to nurses when planning nursing care for their patients. Jordanian and non-Jordanian nurses are required to adjust their caring practices to the cultural and religious needs of Jordanian patients. For example, Islamic dietary law, family ties and kinship, health, and religious activities (fasting and obesity, praying and exercise) need to be incorporated into a nursing model to fit these patients. Furthermore, nurses need to pay attention to gender, identity, roles, communication modes, language, interpersonal relationships, space, the patient's subculture, and the environmental context.

Explanatory Model

The explanatory model developed by Kleinman (1980) and adapted for Arab Muslim nurses perceives health as the spiritual, physical, and psychosocial well-being of individuals (McSweeney, Allen, & Mayo, 1997). Arab Muslim nurses, as well as most Jordanian nurses, have a religiously informed explanatory model that includes these concepts. Spirituality, as grounded in the Muslim worldview, is a theme that is woven throughout Arab culture and nurses' caring. Spirituality is central to the belief system in which spiritual needs take priority over physical needs as a distinctive care pattern. The professional health belief system blends nurses' cultural and religious beliefs, forming a culturally distinct explanation of health beliefs. In other words, in non-Western health contexts, professional models are not dominant but are incorporated into nurses' indigenous worldviews in a way that makes sense within the culture.

CONCEPTS OF ISLAMIC RELIGION RELATED TO THE PRACTICES OF INDIVIDUALS AND HEALTH CARE PROVIDERS

The teachings and law of Islam stem from the *Holy Qur'an* and the *Sunnah* (the speeches of Prophet Mohammad (peace be upon him)). *Tawhid*, which means "the Oneness of Allah," a fundamental in Islam, requires that a Muslim lives in a way that reflects unity of mind and body. Furthermore, tawhid implies that there is no separation of the body from the spiritual dimension of health. The spirituality in an Islamic model is Muslims' inseparability of professional and personal identity. Therefore, any future Arab Muslim nurses' model of care needs to explore spirituality needs and the cultural distinctions that make Arab health care different from the Western nursing tradition.

Islamic teachings inspire Muslims to seek treatment when they get sick. The Prophet Mohammad (peace be upon him) said, seek treatment, because Allah did not send down a sickness but has sent down a medication for it, except for death. However, according to Islamic teachings, mentally competent adult patients have the right to accept or reject treatment. This right does not hold when Islamic rules consider intervention to be obligatory, such as with serious, treatable, infectious disease.

Islam provides dietary rules for Muslims' nutrition. The meat that is allowed (*Halal*) for Muslims must be slaughtered (butchered) in a clearly prescribed way. The dietary guidelines also restrict forbidden foods such as alcohol and pork meat. Breast-feeding is a common practice among Arab and Muslim women. Islam conveys guidelines for Muslim women to breast-feed their babies for up to two years. These guidelines positively correlate with the health of Jordanian mothers and their infants (Jordan Department of Statistics [DOS], 2012).

The Islamic faith has particular rules regarding personal hygiene when going to the toilet. Eating any food while on the toilet is strictly forbidden. Washing one's genitals and hands following going to the toilet is a strict Islamic guideline. Hand washing is also considered fundamental in Islam before praying (along with washing other body parts) and eating.

Privacy and modesty are critical aspects of the Islamic religion. Muslims outside the family are not allowed to touch the opposite sex unless they are married. Muslim women are required to cover their bodies in loose-fitting clothes. It is preferred that Muslim patients should have a health care provider of the same gender. However, a patient is allowed to be cared for by professionals of the opposite sex under certain circumstances, such as emergency cases, the need for the services of a specialist, and the lack of availability of one of the same sex. Whenever a male health care individual provides care for a female patient, a female staff member or a patient's relative should be present. It is important to stress in this context that in Islamic culture, the avoidance of eye contact between opposite genders of patients and health care providers should not be misinterpreted as lack of trust, low self-esteem, or a sign of rejection but as a sign of modesty and humbleness.

The literature reports that female patients prefer female nurses. Women have been found to prefer female nurses for matters of reproductive, sexual health, and intimate or psychosocial issues. Recent research found that in Jordan, gender preferences are stronger among female patients than among male patients (Ahmad & Alasad, 2007). More specifically, 69% of female patients preferred female nurses, whereas only 3.4% preferred male nurses to care for them.

SPECIAL HEALTH PRACTICES FOR ARABS

Muslim patients often seek spiritual and traditional healing practices in addition to modern medicine. Nurses can assist patients in performing some caring action to help spiritual healing, including the recitation of verses of the *Holy Qur'an*, praying, the use of holy water (called *Zamzam*), and a specific repetition of prophetic supplications.

Many individuals, including educated ones, depend on traditional cures and remedies but combine them with modern pharmaceuticals and Western medicine. The traditional healing depends on ancient Arabian therapies that include the use of a variety of plants, herbs, olive oil, honey, black seeds, dates, and special healing methods (Al-Jauziyah, 2003).

The evil eye and *jinn* are supernatural factors in the cultural beliefs as possible causes of illness. Belief in the evil eye as a cause of disease is not limited to the Middle East and North Africa but is also found in parts of Europe (Helman, 2001).

Using specific religious words when providing nursing care is a common practice as a spiritual action that gives confidence in the intervention. For example, saying *Bismallah* (in the name of Allah) before starting any procedure, such as an intravenous infusion or wound dressing, is a caring action that creates rapport between the nurse and patient (Lovering, 2008). Using *Insha Allah* (if Allah's will) comforts the patient, and suggests that his or her condition will improve.

PREMISES IN ISLAM

In addition to those previously mentioned, health care providers should consider the following Islamic premises, obligations, and beliefs when developing care plans:

- Whoever saves a human life saves the life of all human beings (*The Holy Qur'an*).
- Treatment should be sought, for God the Exalted did not create a disease for which He did not create a treatment except senility (Prophet Muhammad PBUH).
- Necessity overrides prohibition.
- The lesser of two harms should be accepted if both cannot be avoided.
- Public interest overrides individual interest.
- Harm has to be removed at all costs if possible.
- A full bath is required after seminal discharge or after menstruation and postnatal bleeding.

- If washing with water or having a bath is not medically advisable or possible, an alternative method of purification, called *Tayammum*, can be performed.
- Muslims are required to pray five times a day.
- Prayers are usually performed on a prayer mat and include various movements such as bowing, prostrating, and sitting.
- It is not necessary for an ill patient to make all the usual prayer movements.
- All types of food are *Halal* (i.e., permissible) in Islam except alcohol and pig products (ham, bacon, pork, pepperoni, salami, etc.).
- Visiting the sick is an important part of a Muslim's duties and is strongly required by Islam.
- Islam stresses respect for all older people.
- Children have a special responsibility to their parents.
- All life is sacred and must be protected.
- Biological life begins at conception.
- The right of the fetus in Islam is similar to the rights of a mature human being: right to life, right of inheritance, right of compensation.
- Islam allows public grief for only three days; this period allows for nonfamily members to visit and offer their condolences. After that period, the family is left to grieve privately.

CONCLUSION

It can be concluded that there are concerns that the existing models and theories of nursing might not fit with other health care systems, specifically those in Jordan. In fact, adopting such theories and models when they are used in isolation from a suitable setting and context could lead to a reinforcement of a traditional health education paradigm. A culturally explicit theory that is underpinned by relevant theoretical constructs is needed to guide the practice and education of nurses in the Arab world.

This chapter discussed inconsistencies between the Western professional nursing vision and Arab Muslim nurses' caring theory; they may be addressed by developing a caring model that reflects the Arab culture and Islamic religious beliefs. Indeed, the number of Arab nursing scholars who completed a Ph.D. degree in nursing from Western countries over the past 20 years is remarkable. These highly prepared scholars are expected to start developing nursing theories that fit the needs of their countries and culture and provide guidelines for nursing education and practice in Arab culture and Islamic communities and for Arab Muslims living abroad. Furthermore, the caring model should provide the basis for an Islamic nursing identity and lead to improving the moral status and image of nursing in the Middle East.

REFERENCES

AbuGharbieh, P., & Suliman, W. (1992). Changing the image of nursing in Jordan through effective role negotiation. *International Nursing Review, 9*(5), 149–152.

Ahmad, M., & Alasad, J. (2007). Patients' preferences for nurses' gender in Jordan. *International Journal of Nursing Practice, 13*, 237–242.

Al-Aitah, R., Cameron, S., Armstrong-Stassen, M., & Horsburgh, M. E. (1999). Effect of gender and education on the quality of nursing work life of Jordanian nurses. *Nursing & Health Care Perspectives, 20*(2), 88–94.

Al-Darazi, F. (2003). Nursing education in the Eastern Mediterranean region: A World Health Organisation initiative. In N. Bryant (Ed.), *Women in nursing in Islamic societies* (pp. 175–187). Oxford: Oxford University Press.

Al-Jauziyah, Q. (2003). *Healing with the medicine of the Prophet (PBUH)*. Riyadh, Saudi Arabia: Darussalam Publications.

Al-Khayat, M. (1997). *Health: An Islamic perspective*. Alexandria, Egypt: World Health Organisation Regional Office for the Eastern Mediterranean Region.

Bryant, N. (2003). *Women in nursing in Islamic societies*. Oxford: Oxford University Press.

Dhami, S., & Sheikh, A. (2008). Health promotion: Reaching ethnic minorities. *Practice Nurse, 36*(8), 21–5.

El-Sanabary, N. (1993). The education and contribution of women health care professionals in Saudi Arabia: The case of nursing. *Social Science Medicine, 37*(11), 1331–1343.

Emami, A., Benner, P., & Ekman, S.-L. (2001). A sociocultural health model for late-in-life immigrants. *Journal of Transcultural Nursing, 12*(1), 15–24.

Harper, M. (2006). Ethical multiculturalism: An evolutionary concept analysis. *Advances in Nursing Science, 29*(2), 110–124.

Helman, C. G. (2001). *Culture, health and illness* (4th ed.). New York: Oxford University Press.

Jan, R. (1996). Rufaidah Al-Asalmiya, the first Muslim nurse. *Image: Journal of Nursing Scholarship, 28*(3), 267–268.

Jordan Department of Statistics (DOS, 2012). *Jordan population and family health survey*. Amman, Jordan: Jordan Department of Statistics.

Jordan Department of Statistics (DOS, 2013). *Kingdom indicators: Statistics*. Amman, Jordan: Jordan Department of Statistics.

Kleinman, A. (1980). *Patients and healers in the context of culture: An exploration of the borderland between anthropology, medicine, and psychiatry*. Berkley, CA: University of California Press.

Leininger, M. (1995). *Transcultural nursing: Concepts, theories, research and practices* (2nd ed.). New York: McGraw-Hill.

Leininger, M. (2002). Part 1. The theory of culture care and ethnonursing research method. In M. Leininger & M. McFarland (Eds.), *Transcultural nursing: Concepts, theories, research & practice* (3rd ed.) (pp. 71–98). New York: McGraw-Hill.

Leininger, M., & McFarland, M. R. (2002). *Transcultural nursing: concepts, theories, research, and practice* (3rd ed.). New York: McGraw-Hill.

Lovering, S. (2008). *Arab Muslim nurses' experience of the meaning of caring*. [Online] Available from http://www.researchgate.net/publication/265079901_Arab_Muslim_Nurses%27_Experiences_Of_The_Meaning_Of_Caring

McSweeney, J., Allen, J., & Mayo, K. (1997). Exploring the use of explanatory models in nursing research and practice. *Image: International Journal of Nursing Scholarship, 29*(3), 243–248.

Nydell, M. K. (2005). *Understanding Arabs: A guide for modern times*. Boston: Intercultural Press.

Rassool, H. (2004). Commentary: An Islamic perspective. *Journal of Advanced Nursing*, *46*(3), 281.

Retso, J. (2002). *Arabs in antiquity: Their history from the Assyrians to the Umayyads*. London and New York: Routledge.

Wehbe-Alamah, H. (2005). *Generic and professional health care beliefs, expressions & practices of Syrian Muslims living in the mid-western United States*. Unpublished doctoral dissertation, Duquesne University, Pittsburg, Pennsylvania.

Wehbe-Alamah, H. (2008). Bridging generic and professional care practices for Muslim patients through the use of Leininger's culture care modes. *Contemporary Nurse*, *28*(1–2), 83–97.

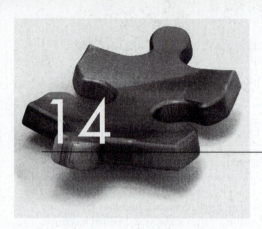

Mexico: Nursing Theory, Research, and Education

Esther C. Gallegos and Bertha Cecilia Salazar-González

INTRODUCTION

The use of nursing theories in Mexico began in the academic sector. However, despite being strongly influenced by the nursing approach in the United States through the use of textbooks published in English, theoretical content from these sources was incorporated into the various courses that are part of the curriculum for both undergraduate and graduate nursing when the latter studies in nursing began to emerge as a field of study within the Country (the 1980s).

As in other Latin American countries, nursing in Mexico developed in the heart of medical sciences and evolved to form the theoretical basis for nursing's professional mission. The implementation of social security brought great medical specialization (primarily oriented to the biological aspects of disease) and the construction of large hospitals across Mexico. Nursing became an administrative function that facilitated hospital operations and moved away from the patient's bedside. In response to the introduction of advanced medical technology, post-technical specialty programs, such as intensive care, pediatrics, surgery, the administration of services, and operating room nursing, were created. These specialty programs addressed the demand for health care support and hospital management. Unfortunately, patients' needs for comprehensive nursing care were virtually unmet.

Although nursing care in health institutions was and remains governed primarily as executants of medical prescriptions, and administrator's
176

decisions (providing more of a hotel-type service than care management), the training process for nurses has created its own theoretical and methodological concepts within the discipline. Theoretical aspects from theorists such as Orem (2001), Roy & Andrews (1991; 1999), Roy (2009), King (1981), and Neuman and Fawcett (2011), among others, have been included in nursing courses without reducing the high content of medical sciences and minor social sciences in the curriculum. The adoption of the *nursing care process* (or simply *nursing process* [NP]) as the systematic method for planning and processing comprehensive care for people with a health–disease status reflected the way nurses used to learn about their patients (Secretaría de Salud [Mexican Secretariat of Health, or SSA in Spanish], 2011).

From nursing's formalization as a profession in 1905, until the early 1950s, the medical model prevailed both in nursing education and practice. Within this period of time, the hospital's delivered care system was based on diagnosing and treating diseases; providing hygiene and comfort to those receiving nursing care was considered to be a distinct field of professional nursing for individuals hospitalized by certain diseases (Rosales-Barrera & Gómez-Reyes, 2004).

Use of Theory in Nursing Delivery Systems

In Mexico, the provision of health services is carried out by social security (Instituto Mexicano del Seguro Social [IMSS], and Instituto de Seguridad y Servicios Sociales para los Trabajadores del Estado [ISSSTE]), the government (Secretaría de Salud y Asistencia [SSA]), and private health care, three subsystems that differ substantially. Each of these subsystems of nursing is based according to its philosophy, goals, and organizational structures. However, seven years ago, the directors of nursing of health institutes, nursing professors, and researchers associated with the federal government's nursing headquarters formed the Permanent Committee of Nursing (CPE in Spanish). This organization generates national standards about what nurses are and should do to address the population's health needs. Nursing leaders are still involved in the three subsystems, and the CPE's recommendations apply to both social security and private health care.

One of this committee's main achievements is the development of nursing care plans (NCPs) that delineate the *what to do* of nursing. Two publications available to Mexican nursing professionals have introduced 40 NCP plans (described in terms of medical diagnosis and treatment) that affect an individual upon entering a health facility or receiving outpatient care at it (Secretaría de Salud [Health Secretariat],

2012, 2013). The theoretical foundation of these plans comprises the diagnostic procedures from the North American Nursing Diagnosis Association (NANDA), the Nursing Interventions Classification (NIC), and the Nursing Outcomes Classification (NOC).

In the context of *inpatients*, nursing care plans apply to all people who require hospitalization as a result of a self-care deficit diagnosis. Hygiene and patient comfort are the basis of a diagnosis within the context of the *self-care deficit nursing theory* discussed subsequently and considers two actions required before interventions:

1. Verify the patient's ability to exercise independent self-care.
2. Observe the patient's need for hygienic activities.

Primary care (community and outpatient clinics) handle prevention and health promotion. The NCPs applied at the primary care level include diagnoses expressed with self-care deficits nursing theory (SCDNT) concepts. The *self-care deficit in personal hygiene* and the *feeding deficit* NCPs apply to patients with a permanent intravenous catheter and those suffering from chronic renal failure, respectively, and are managed on an outpatient basis. The NCPs regarding *willingness to improve self-care* and *willingness to improve nutrition* are for individuals with cardiovascular risk and obesity, respectively. Interventions identified for these diagnoses emphasize education, information, and guidance from the nurse. The application of NCPs occurs mainly in hospitals and premiere clinics that belong to the Secretariat of Health at the federal and state levels. These institutions grant health services to those without social security health care benefits, generally the most vulnerable sector of the population.

The concept of what the nursing profession is and what it should do in private hospitals has evolved. After a number of years of considering NP "the core of nursing knowledge," nurses from private hospitals (Hospital Angeles, n. d.) recognized that sustaining their professional interventions by applying the nursing process was not enough to advance the profession. They realized the need to strengthen the theory behind and to adopt forms of care that were grounded in scientific evidence. These colleagues understood that the model of care applied until the early 21st century reduced people to a biological dimension, neglecting psychological and sociocultural processes that play a role in human well-being that is as—or more—important than the pathophysiological processes emphasized by the medical model. These nurses realized they needed to better understand the interplay between physiological, psychological, and sociocultural variables to provide comprehensive care that supports the essence of the profession.

Based on this reasoning, nurses restructured the nursing model to incorporate theoretical and methodological elements in the formulation and operation of care. Patient needs are determined along two dimensions. First, needs are identified according to Henderson's theory (1978) regarding health, care, person, and environment, and to Orem's concepts (2001): self-care and self-care agency. Nursing diagnoses are based on NANDA taxonomy (2011). A care plan is designed next and managed according to the nursing systems *middle-range theory*, which establishes both the structure and content of nursing care. The results of the care provided are quantified in terms of patient satisfaction and are monitored via the outcome standards defined by a hospital's nursing group.

The second source to identify patients' needs come from the medical treatment in the form of pharmacological prescriptions, diet, and others, which are integrated into the nursing care plan. In this case, results are evaluated in terms of treatment accomplishment: the patient receives the prescribed treatment in the appropriate dose and method and as scheduled. The content of the nursing model followed in private hospitals reflects the integration of the care derived from medical treatment and the comprehensive assessment performed by nursing professionals.

OREM'S *SELF-CARE DEFICIT NURSING THEORY*

In the last three decades, a number of investigations in Mexico have used the concepts of Orem. Orem's (2001) *self-care deficit theory* explains what nursing is and identifies when nursing care is needed. The theory has six main concepts: self-care (or dependent care), self-care agency, therapeutic self-care demand, self-care deficit, nursing agency and basic conditioning factors.

Orem (2001) theorizes that all individuals need actions—usually more than one self-care activity to be performed at a certain time and place, constituting the self-care demand (SCD)—to care for their health; to develop such actions, individuals need special capabilities, such as to interpret levels of blood glucose when checking it by themselves; when the SCD is higher than the capabilities a self-care deficit occurs. *Nurse agency*— which is nurses professional ability developed through special training— is required only when a self-care deficit is present.

Certain factors internal or external to an individual affect self-care activities; these are basic conditioning factors modifying positively or negatively self-care activities and abilities. Orem (2001) proposed that the *basic conditioning factors* include age, gender, developmental state, health state, family system, sociocultural orientation, patterns of living, environment, and resource adequacy. These factors can also apply to nursing agency.

Self-care and self-care agency are determined by self-care needs, which are the reason for performing self-care and developing self-care agency. The three types of *self-care requisites* are universal, developmental, and health deviational. Conceptualizations of these three types of needs constitute the framework within which self-care and self-care agency work.

Three *middle-range theories* are derived from the general self-care deficit nursing theory: *self-care, self-care deficit*, and *nursing system. Self-care theory* explains it as a human regulatory function; The self-care deficit theory explains why a person needs or requires nursing care; and the nursing system describes the structure of the nursing practice.

The theoretical basis of nursing care in health institutions focuses predominantly on medical and organizational knowledge whereas the theoretical content of the professional nursing curriculum focuses on medical sciences; nursing theory; and social, instrumental, or methodological sciences. These two approaches—(a) nursing care based on the medical model in health institutions and (b) organizational knowledge with limited nursing theory content in education—have been maintained in parallel so that this mixture of disciplines equally supports nursing education and nursing practice.

It should be noted that the content of nursing theories originates not from original publications by diverse authors such as Orem, Roy, and Pender but from secondary sources (e.g., Mariner-Tomey & Alligood, 2008) that summarize and often interpret a theory according to particular contexts, reducing—and possibly skewing—the universality of the theoretical knowledge.

Theories Used in Nursing Models

When new graduates from programs that teach comprehensive nursing enter the workforce, they must perform according to the career profiles demanded by the health institutions that employ them. They leave behind what they learned about theory-supported care in their degree programs. The content of nursing theories and how they are incorporated into nursing education, practice, and research in Mexico must be understood within these dichotomous perspectives. According to some published (and unpublished) literature, the most commonly used models are Orem's *general theory of self-care (2001)*, The Roy's *adaptation model (2009)*, and Pender's *health promotion model (2002)*, among others. The use of these theories is increasingly based more on concepts and their interrelationships with specific populations such as adults with diabetes type 2, community dwelling elders and youth.

Research Related to Orem's Theories   Nursing theory is primarily used in research. Models and theories such as those by Orem (2001), Roy (2009), Neuman and Fawcett (2011), and Pender (2002) are often discussed in articles and theses. The following paragraphs describe studies including concepts developed by Orem and Roy. Many of these studies were performed by graduate students in nursing, but few of them have been published. A review of the published reports and gray literature (unpublished) shows that some of them refer to Orem's concepts but have different variables. Some of these concepts have been implemented in interventions and have generated middle-range theories that complement, or deepen, Orem's theories applying knowledge from other disciplines such as psychology, sociology, among others. Some of the conducted research have been integrated into and summarized in descriptive, correlational, and intervention studies.

Self-Care Concepts

As mentioned before, the central concepts of the *self-care deficit nursing theory* (Orem, 2001) include self-care (dependent care), self-care agency (dependent self-care agency), therapeutic self-care demand, self-care deficit, nursing agency, and basic conditioning factors. *Self-care requisite* is defined as a subconcept and sometimes is included in research studies.

Self-care is one concept that has been described verbally by patient groups. A first example is the work reported by Méndez-Salazar, Becerril-Estrada, Morales-Pilar, and Pérez-Ilagor (2010) from in-depth interviews with older people (n = 10) diagnosed with type 2 diabetes mellitus (T2DM). In that population, self-care involves oral hygiene, eating a balanced diet, exercising, and periodically checking lower extremities and monitoring glucose levels and body changes caused by or associated with chronic disease.

In a second example, self-care agency was defined (Gallegos, Cárdenas, & Salas, 1999) according to interviews with patients with T2DM. The interview content was analyzed qualitatively for subsequent categorization according to the dimensions identified by Backscheider (as cited in Orem, 2001). The final categories included lifestyle, physical functioning, and attitude. From these dimensions a questionnaire composed by 15 items, Likert-type responses were generated.

A third example shows the use of self-care requisites to guide the development of self-care agency in adults with T2DM. Using educational sessions with procedure demonstrations, Medellín-Vélez (2007) facilitated the development and application of self-care skills in adults diagnosed with T2DM to satisfy the universal self-care requisites (sufficient intake of air, water and food, elimination, balance between activity and rest, between solitude and social interaction, prevention of hazards, and promotion of human functioning) and the pharmacological treatment requirements (self-care requisites derived from chronic disease).

Relationships Between Concepts   Studies that related to the concepts of the self-care nursing theory were the most abundant in the literature. Most of the schemata used explained self-care activities as the *outcome*, the *self-care agency* as the mediator concept, and *basic conditioning factors* as the independent variable(s) that directly affected self-care agency and self-care through self-care agency. The studies discussed next followed this schemata of relationships.

Maya-Morales and Fonseca-Castaño (2008) reported a significant positive relationship between family support (defined as the *basic conditioning factor*) and self-care in patients with T2DM. In similar research, Hernández-Méndez, Martínez-González, and Landeros-Olvera (2009) found that age, sex, marital status, and education (also defined as basic conditioning factors) explained 25% of the variance in self-care agency in patients with hypertension. Compeán-Ortiz, Gallegos-Cabriales, González-González, and Gómez-Meza (2010) reported a low level of self-care (SC) in adults with T2DM that explained glycosylated hemoglobin (HbA1c), body mass index (BMI), and body fat levels of 9–41%. Landeros and Gallegos (2005) used an open population for research on the predictive ability of perceived health status (i.e., basic conditioning factors measured as health state perception by the Medical outcome study, short form questionnaire [MOS-SF] and self-care agency); the adjusted $R^2 = 0.09$ was low as was the self-care agency average.

In correlational studies, Bañuelos and Gallegos (2001) hypothesized that basic conditioning factors influenced self-care agency in the same way that they influenced self-care in older adults. They further assumed that glycemic control, indicated by HbA1c, would be affected by self-care. This hypothesis was confirmed by using a multiple regression model in which 14.2% of the HbA1c variance was explained by self-care agency, self-care, and the basic conditioning factors.

Research studies correlating self-care deficit nursing theory concepts that pose *middle-range theories* for specific groups that are in a temporary or permanent state of compromised health are beginning to circulate. These studies are often found among theses of students pursuing a master's degree of science in nursing. Sánchez-Meza (2012) designed the middle-range theory of T2DM-dependent care that was derived from the middle-range theory of self-care deficit (Orem, 2001, 146–147). Dependent care provided by the caregiver is influenced by his/her abilities (dependent care agency), which in turn are impacted by health status, age, gender, occupation, education, and knowledge about T2DM (all defined as basic conditioning factors). Of the dependent care attributed primarily to women (85%), 29.8% was explained by the basic conditioning factors and the dependent care agency, both being highly significant (β = .557, p = .001).

Intervention Studies   Vicente-Ruiz (2006) addressed the problem of an increase in sedentary behavior and consumption of energy-dense food among adolescents. The middle-range theory of preventive self-care of T2DM for adolescents at risk was derived from Orem's middle-range theory self-care deficit, incorporating knowledge on diet and physical activity at the adolescent stage that were inherent to self-care. Concepts that were related included perceived health status (defined as a basic conditioning factor), self-efficacy, productive capacity (defined as a self-care agency), diet, and physical activity (defined as self-care actions). The response variables included insulin resistance (IR), BMI, waist circumference, body composition (BC), and lipid profile. A 12-week controlled intervention to increase physical activity and decrease the consumption of foods with a high fat content was developed.

Various analyses showed a significant effect of the intervention on the increase in self-care agency: (a) Partial analyses showed the predictive ability of the perceived health and social support (defined as basic conditioning factors) for self-care agency, explaining 21% of its variance. (b) *Self-care*, defined in this case as a calorie consumption that matches calorie expenditure, should improve as a result of the increase in the intervention's self-care agency. In fact, this expectation was supported by the decrease in BMI, BC, and (LDL). Importantly, self-care (mainly food consumption) significantly predicted 44% of the homeostatic model assessment (HOMA) index values, an indicator of insulin resistance (IR).

To improve metabolic control in adults with T2DM, Gallegos, Ovalle-Berúmen, and Gómez-Meza (2006) developed an 18-month controlled intervention consisting of education and individualized counseling for patients receiving outpatient treatment. The middle-range theory of self-care deficit formed the theoretical basis and included the self-care agency and self-care concepts; adaptation and environmental barriers were also considered as basic conditioning factors affecting the self-care agency. The outcome variable was HbA1c; the experimental and control groups were equivalent in terms of factors that affect glycemic control such as age, education, BMI, years with T2DM, and HbA1c, which were considered basic conditioning factors. The intervention in the experimental group was effective in reducing HbA1c but not self-care; the explained variance in HbA1c figures was 21.5% for self-care agency, environmental barriers, and the interaction of self-care agency with adaptation. Self-care scores for the experimental and control groups did not show a significant difference; 34.2% was explained by self-care agency, environmental barriers, and the interaction of self-care agency with adaptation.

Nursing *Theories with Concepts from Other Disciplines*

The phenomenon of childhood obesity and its control constitutes a public health problem in Mexico. The development of obesity is complex with various intervening factors that require a multidisciplinary approach for study. One study performed by Ph.D. students in nursing science addressed this phenomenon using concepts from Orem's self-care deficit and from Bronfenbrenner's (1981) bioecological theory of human development to build the middle-range theory of environmental and familial factors in the development of cardiometabolic risk factors in school-aged children (Bañuelos-Barrera, 2011).

Bronfenbrenner (1981) theorizes that individuals develop within ecological strata among themselves. These strata conform to a concentric structure from inside to outside (microsystems, mesosystem, exosystem, and macrosystem), meaning the closest environment to the individual (microsystem) to the farthest in the individuals' daily living (macrosystem). This theoretical structure was used to situate Orem's interrelated concepts in the central stratum and the school environment in the following stratum.

The microsystem was based on concepts concerning children's actions related to eating patterns and physical activity, representing self-care, and mothers' dependent care agency in handling the eating patterns and physical activity of their children that are basic conditioning factors of family health and personal mother–child factors and family atmosphere. The mesosystem was the school environment. The resulting variable was the level of cardiometabolic risk such as BMI, acanthosis nigricans, lipids, and C-reactive protein. The model is represented in Figure 14–1.

The middle-range theory involved environmental and family factors in the development of cardiometabolic risk factors in school children.

Results confirmed that self-care activities of the school-aged child were explained by 34% of the variables defined as microsystem components whereas the cardiometabolic risk factors—HDLc 13%, LDLc 2%, and body fat 10% were explained by components of the micro- and mesosystems.

Research developed by Gutiérrez-Valverde (2010) approached the identification of a framework to assess risk for developing T2DM in adults from three theoretical perspectives: (a) Orem's self-care deficit theory,

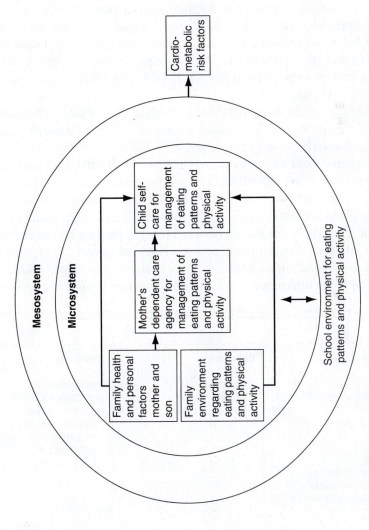

FIGURE14–1 Environmental and family factors in the development of cardiometabolic risk factors in school children

(b) a construct of the model gene-environment interaction (Hernández, Blazer, 2006), and (c) clinical knowledge about the inheritance of T2DM. Based on these perspectives, the author identified the middle-range theory of T2DM risk levels in individuals with genetic heritage.

The gene-environment construct, was represented by the basic conditioning factors, including familial and environmental systems. Operational definition for family system, was familial aggregation, and for environmental factors, socioeconomic status and years of education. Exposure to or risk behavior accompanied the self-care concept and included eating patterns and physical activity. The outcome variable was health status defined as indicators or phenotypes for T2DM. The middle-range theory is presented in Figure 14–2.

Participants in the study T2DM risk levels in individuals with genetic heritage, were members of 37 families who were contacted through a relative who had been previously diagnosed with T2DM. With the addition of other family members who may or may not have had chronic disease, the participants totaled 207 individuals (n = 99 diagnosed with T2DM, n = 71 without T2DM). Analyses showed a partial effect of basic conditioning factors (physical activity) on self-care, explaining 26.3% of its variation. A significant interaction was shown between level of poverty and education, meaning that years of education depends on level of poverty; also years of education in conjunction with family system variables explained 18.6% of the variance in the difference in kilocalories consumed minus expenditure.

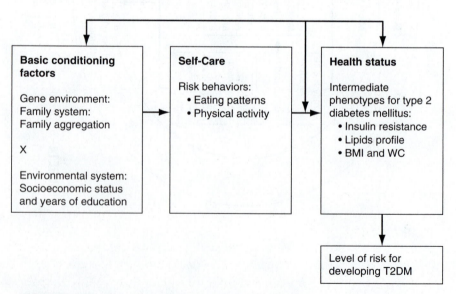

FIGURE14–2   Middle-Range Theory: Risk Factors for T2DM in Individuals with Genetic Inheritance

The predictive ability of the variables of education, aggregation of hypertension, and obesity on risk factors for T2DM on the subgroup of participants without T2DM was determined. These three variables explained the variance of total cholesterol concentration (42%), triglycerides (28%), and the HOMA index (23%).

Results of this research showed utility-applying constructs and concepts from non nursing fields of knowledge, such as genetic and environmental sciences to nursing theories as Orem's self-care deficit.

Orem's general theory of self-care deficit is one of the most frequently mentioned theories in the Mexican nursing community. Among the concepts that integrate theory, self-care, self-care agency, and basic conditioning factors are those most often used in adults with diabetes type 2 and comorbidities such as hypertension; these three concepts also are fundamental to explaining the effect of self-care actions in diminishing metabolic risk factors. Less frequently used concepts corresponded to universal self-care requisites such as nutritional and physical activity requirements and balancing rest and activity. Other nursing constructs such as nursing care systems, particularly educational support, are frequently reported as interventions that seek to improve self-care agency and self-care.

Participants in various studies included groups recruited because of a particular common health or well being characteristic. These characteristics made up groups of seniors, adults with T2DM complications, adults with obesity or CVD, inpatients, postpartum women with hypertension; also, groups of participants were comprised by healthy people recruited at their homes through geographic sampling. The researchers, whose investigations were summarized previously, considered the availability of culturally appropriate instruments for the study population, which is one of the most challenging problems when consolidating research in nursing theory.

The summarized studies show empirically verified relationships among self-care deficit nursing theory concepts that contribute to the self-care theory's credibility. Explanatory or predictive relationships were demonstrated for basic conditioning factors on self-care, self-care agency on self-care, educational interventions, and counseling on the operation of self-care agency and increased self-care. The most frequently used basic conditioning factors corresponded to characteristics and individuals' perceptions such as age, sex, health status, and knowledge followed by factors associated with individual or family livelihood, such as socioeconomic stratum and education. Self-care agency and self-care are geared toward disease or disease risk factors. It should be noted that a relationship between self-care and results that indicate health status as in the case of biochemical measurements in T2DM (e.g., HbA1c) has not been consistently demonstrated.

RESEARCH GUIDED BY ROY'S ADAPTATION MODEL

In academia, Roy's *adaptation model* (Roy & Andrews, 1991, 1999; Roy, 2009) is considered important and uses a theoretical basis of research. Two nursing schools, Universidad Autónoma de San Luís Potosí and Universidad de Guanajuato, reported the use of Roy's theory by graduate students conducting research work. However, in some reports, it is not clear whether the source used is the original version of Roy's model or that of a secondary source, such as Marriner-Tomey & Alligood, (2008) because some published research papers do not document the use of the model or provide conceptual-operational definitions consistent with those established by Roy. No published information on the use of Roy's model in nursing practice or education has been found.

Roy's adaptation model (2009) views persons as human adaptive systems exposed to internal and external stimuli. According to Roy's adaptation model, stimuli (focal, contextual, or residual) activate coping processes (regulator and cognator) to generate responses through four adaptive modes: physiological, self-concept, interdependent, and role function. Although the proposed model does not provide a direct relationship between stimuli and adaptive responses, Roy notes that a given stimulus can affect more than one mode (Roy, 2009, p. 45); therefore, the study of direct relationships between stimuli and modes or responses is relevant.

In academia, Roy's adaptation model serves as the parent theory used to formulate particular theories or situation specific theories (Meleis, 2012) to guide research. Strategies suggested for theory formalization by Fawcett (1999) are used to analyze congruence between proposed concepts and their respective parent constructs to be tested in descriptive or intervention studies.

In Mexico, Roy's adaptation model has been used to describe the physiological mode in older adults with hypertension (Esquivel-Rodríguez & García Campos, 2007) and in patients with peritoneal dialysis (Alarcón-Rosales, 2007). Roy's model has also been used to study the relationships between the model's concepts: stimuli and the four modes in cancer patients receiving chemotherapy (García-Valenzuela, Cuevas-Cansino, Tinoco-López, 2004), and between contextual stimuli and self-concept mode in women who had suffered mastectomy (Bañuelos-Barrera P., Bañuelos Barrera, Y., Esquivel-Rodríguez, & Moreno-Avila, 2007).

Research related to Roy's (1999; 2009) adaptation model in graduate nursing at the Autonomous University of Nuevo León has been descriptive and interventional. Relationships between variables that served as stimuli and coping processes (cognator or regulator) have been tested, but very few studies explored relationships between coping processes and adaptive responses. Intervention studies guided by Roy's (1999; 2009) model have shown the significant effects of interventions, and some have addressed the relationship between contextual stimuli and adaptive responses. The descriptive and intervention studies will be described in the following paragraphs.

Descriptive T2DM Studies

Roy's adaptation model allows the introduction of concrete related concepts to represent focal and contextual stimuli, coping processes (cognator and regulator), and modes or adaptive responses (physiological, self-concept, interdependence, and role function). Roy (2009) notes that at some point, a response can become a stimulus; therefore, the model is flexible. The following paragraphs describe the results and concepts used in three studies.

Two descriptive studies on people with T2DM (Lazcano-Ortíz & Salazar-González, 2009; Castro-Espinoza, 2012) were conducted, and another focused on an elderly population (Kantún-Marín, 2012). The research work by Lazcano-Ortíz and Salazar-González (2009) found that stress was used as a contextual stimulus and was negatively related to coping processes; stress accounted for 51% of the variance in coping processes; for each unit of increasing stress, coping processes declined .57. However, perceived stress was not associated with physiological adaptation, as indicated by HbA1c, cholesterol, triglycerides, and body mass index and was negatively related to psychosocial adaptation as measured by the Psychosocial Adjustment to Illness Scale (PAIS) of Derogatis (1985). For each unit of increase in stress, psychosocial adaptation decreased .47; the explained variance was 28%. Coping processes did not mediate among contextual stimulus, stress, and psychosocial adaptation (role responses, self-concept, and interdependence) or quality of life that represented general adaptation (Lazcano-Ortíz & Salazar González, 2009). Stress is known to have an impact on glucose levels; however, the study did not observe this effect.

The descriptive-correlational research conducted by Castro-Espinoza (2012) reports that years following a T2DM diagnosis (contextual stimulus) and insulin levels (regulatory process) contributed to 9.6% and 68.5% of the explained variance of Hb1Ac and the HOMA index, respectively. Compliance with medications was negatively associated with coping processes; health status (focal) was positively associated with coping processes as measured by Roy's scale (Gutiérrez-López, et al. 2007). However, compliance with medications and health status were not associated with insulin levels, which appears to confirm that disease degeneration continues to run its course despite medical treatment and health perception.

In her dissertation, Kantún-Marín (2012) used a multivariate analysis to show a relationship between the self-perception of aging and the environmental characteristics used as focal stimuli on executive function and intrapsychic factors (cognator). Physical activity was related to the mechanisms of functional performance and executive function. Of the variance in executive function, perception of aging and environmental characteristics explained 24%; depression symptoms explained 24%; 4% explained intrapsychic mechanisms; and 4% explained functional performance mechanisms.

In Kantún-Marín's (2012) study, multivariate models included two focal stimuli (self-perception of aging and environmental characteristics) and two contextual stimuli (physical activity and depressive symptoms) as independent variables, and the dependent variables of perception of physical health, life satisfaction, and sociability showed significance for all models. Post hoc univariate analysis found that 18% of the variance was explained by physical health, 30% by life satisfaction, and 35% by sociability (adaptive responses).

A third model in the Kantún-Marín (2012) study showed that coping processes represented by intrapsychic factors and executive function are related to adaptive modes represented by physical health, life satisfaction, and sociability. The explained variance of perceived physical health was 7%; of life satisfaction, 25%; and of sociability, 15%. The mechanisms of functional performance did not show significance. This is the only study that has tested relationships between stimuli and coping processes, between stimuli and adaptive responses, and between coping processes and adaptive responses (Kantún-Marín, 2012).

Intervention Studies

An intervention study conducted by Villarreal-Reyna (2006) was guided by Roy's (1998; 2009) adaptation model and developed to test positive adaptation of attitude toward caregiving, anxiety, and humor of people caring for a relative with Alzheimer's disease. Between psico-educative sessions and as part of the intervention, caregivers were assigned several tasks to improve their attitudes and humor regarding their caregiving. The study showed significantly improving positive attitude toward care and reduced bad humor and anxiety immediately after the intervention and one month later. Completion of assigned tasks to reduce caregivers' bad humor was correlated to their baseline attitude and anxiety (Villarreal-Reyna, 2006).

Quasiexperimental studies have been conducted on exercise intervention in people with type 2 diabetes (T2DM), elderly people, and young women who are obese and overweight. All participants achieved improvements of the variables (Cruz-Quevedo, 2006; Landeros-Olvera, 2010; Muñoz-Canché, 2001). However, only the Muñoz-Canché study verified the effect of contextual stimuli on response variables, which were not significant.

Lazcano-Ortiz and Salazar-González (2008) validated the adaptation scale and coping processes in people with T2DM. Factor extraction identified six factors, one more than suggested by Roy. The factors accounted for 65.29% of the total variance in the scale. The Cronbach coefficient of internal consistency was 0.93. García-Valenzuela et al. (2004) report that they designed an instrument for assessing physiological and role representation modes; however, they do not provide data on its development or validation.

The way in which Roy's model has been applied in research provides a broad view of biological and psychosocial variables representative of the entire human being. The following relationships provide credibility to this model (Castro-Espinoza, 2012; Kantún-Marín, 2012; Landeros-Olvera, 2010; Lazcano-Ortíz & Salazar-González, 2009; Villarreal-Reyna, 2006). Focal stimuli (such as years with T2DM, perceived health status, and aging) and contextual factors (such as stress, intrapsychic aspects, functional performance mechanisms, anxiety, and executive function) have explained coping processes and adaptation levels indicated by biochemical fractions in metabolic control, psychosocial adaptation, quality of life, and use of humor. Two exercise interventions representing contextual stimuli improved levels of adiponectine, leptin, percentage of body fat, representing physiologic mode and physical self-concept of young women with overweight and obesity (Landeros-Olvera, 2010); a resistance exercise training used a focal stimuli was able to show decrease percentage of glycated hemoglobin and improved muscle strength representing the physiologic mode and self-concept (physical self) in adults with DMT2 (Muñoz-Canché, 2001). These results relate to Roy's (2009, p. 45) notation that a given stimulus can affect more than one mode.

THEORY USED IN NURSING EDUCATION PROGRAMS

Most undergraduate curricula in Mexican nursing schools integrate courses in medical sciences, psychosocial studies, methodology, and nursing. The theoretical content of nursing courses includes elements of nursing theories without necessarily transferring them to clinical or community practice. What underpins student practice are diagnoses based on NANDA (2011) classification, or Gordon's (1987) functional health patterns.

The textbook *Nursing Models and Theories* (Spanish version) by Marriner-Tomey and Alligood (2008) is used to teach nursing theories. These authors summarize the biographical aspects of the theorists such as Meleis (2012), Orem (2001), Roy (2009), Henderson (1978), among others, and describe general theories with some simplified definitions of concepts. In general and exclusively as an academic exercise, the textbook formulates care plans using each of the theorists' directions for applying the theory. The current nursing practice in health institutions, which often does not coincide with the theoretical perspective, highly influences students' clinical and community practice.

Nursing curricula that explicitly include only one nursing theory are the exception. One exception is a program that uses Watson's (2008) theory of human caring as the support that guides the content and development in academic programs. Its inclusion in courses such as the science of human caring and of human caring in adults shows how the theory of human caring permeates undergraduate nursing curriculum. Professional master's degree programs (similar in scope to nurse practitioner certification) offered by nursing schools are guided by Watson's theoretical framework. Qualitative phenomenology and microethnography, among others, are advocated as research methods. Master's students of the program based on Watson's theory, apply model proposals of care that focus on humanizing nursing care for specific groups; the most commonly applied research design is uncontrolled intervention.

CONCLUSION

The health–disease problems prevalent in Mexico produce nursing care needs, and those who suffer must be analyzed in a context much broader than the physical dimension alone. Individual, group, and social responses to disease as well as risk factors for developing it are better explained when the myriad of possible human responses facing aggressions are considered. These responses for coping with health problems differ according to the sociocultural differences of various populations.

The current situation in Mexico reflected in epidemiological reports places a priority on chronic degenerative diseases and violence leading to the disintegration of the social fabric by breaking family ties and geographically displacing affected groups.

Social, economic and political problems or risk situations that affect individuals, families, and groups do not necessarily differ from the biological and psychological issues that affect their health status as in hypertension, depression, among others. However, the interaction between the biological dimensions and sociopolitical, cultural, and economic factors favors highly complex health problems, making practically useless the traditional diagnoses made via physical, psychological, and social domains. Considering excess variables when trying to explain or understand a health–disease problem provides substantial methodological difficulties. Therefore, envisioning models and more comprehensive theories can extend and deepen the intricate relationships between an individual and the environment.

Health–disease problems in Mexico remain present and increase daily, compromising the well-being and quality of life of individuals, families, and society. Obesity, T2DM, cardiovascular disease (CVD), and cancer are associated with habits such as eating an unhealthy diet, leading a sedentary lifestyle, and having little access to preventive and curative medicine. Access to health services is determined by families' economic capacity and/or by the stable employment of the head of household in the productive sector, a condition that enables these families to rely on health care provided by social security. In the absence of stable employment status, family members receive health services from government institutions, which often do not have sufficient resources to meet the high demand generated by chronic degenerative diseases. These eligibility conditions are determined by the Mexican government's health and social policies.

The research studies described in this chapter were guided by various theories and show mostly interest on individuals, placing elements of the family and social environment peripherally. The interventions discussed include factors that have theoretically been identified as causes that need to be modified (such as behavior, attitude, and knowledge). Although the theoretical frameworks (Orem and Roy) have proven to be useful, they are clearly limited to the study of individual or family behavior. It is necessary to visualize a theory that, in addition to treating the individual, explain its structure and predicts the relationships, interactions, and mediations of other factors that emphasize unhealthy behaviors leading to overt disease, malaise, and poor quality of life.

At the individual level, it is also necessary to extend the scope and type of variables that are known to be directly or indirectly responsible for an outcome variable, whether it is behavior, attitude, or something else in addition to the extension of other measurements. Scientific advancements are revealing a series of connections at the level of molecules, and biochemical, physical, and electric signalizations that not only affect the individual's physiological, genetic, and neurological processes but also associate phenotypes with feelings, perceptions, and behaviors. This consideration is akin to understanding nursing as the diagnosis and treatment of human responses to health and disease; however, it does not explicitly reflect contextual factors.

In sum, nursing theory should provide the structure to explain comprehensively health-related problems of complex individuals who are parts of families and social groups and interact in different environments that are directly and indirectly responsible for their health status.

REFERENCES

Alarcón-Rosales. (2007). Modelo de adaptación: aplicación en pacientes con diálisis perito-neal continua ambulatoria. [Adaptation Model: Application in patients with ambulatory continuous peritoneal dialysis]. *Revista de Enfermería del Instituto Mexicano del Seguro Social, 15*(3), 155–130.

Bañuelos-Barrera, P., & Gallegos, E. C. (2001). Autocuidado y control en adultos mayores con diabetes [Self-care and control in older adults with diabetes]. *Desarrollo Científico de Enfermería, 9*(4), 100–106.

Bañuelos-Barrera, P., Bañuelos-Barrera, Y., Esquivel-Rodríguez, M., & Moreno-Avila, V. (2007). Autoncepto de mujeres con cáncer en mama. [Self-concept of women with breast cancer]. *Revista de Enfermería del Seguro Social, 15*(3), 129–134.

Bañuelos-Barrera, Y. (2011). Factores ambientales y familiares en el desarrollo de riesgo cardiometabólico en niños de edad escolar. Tesis de Doctoral no publicada, Universidad Autónoma de Nuevo León-Facultad de Enfermería. [Family and environmental factors in the development of cardiometabolic risk in school-aged children. Unpublished thesis, Autonomous University of Nuevo Leon, School of Nursing, Monterrey, Mexico].

Bronfrenbrenner, U. (1981). *The ecology of human development: Experiments by nature and design.* Harvard University Press.

Castro-Espinoza, J. M. (2012). Adaptación fisiológica en personas viviendo con diabetes tipo 2. Tesis doctoral inédita, Universidad Autónoma de Nuevo León-Facultad de Enfermería. [Physiological adaptation in people living with type 2 diabetes. Unpublished doctoral dissertation, Autonomous University of Nuevo Leon, School of Nursing, Monterrey, México].

Compeán-Ortiz, L. G., Gallegos-Cabriales, E. C., González-González, J. G., & Gómez-Meza, M. V. (2010). Conductas de autocuidado eindicadores de salud en adultos con diabetes tipo 2. [Self-care behaviors and health indicators in adults with type 2 diabetes]. *Revista Latino-Americana de Enfermagem, 18*(4), 675–680.

Cruz-Quevedo, J. E. (2006). Ejercicio de resistencia muscular en la funcionalidad física del adultos mayor. Tesis doctoral inédita, Universidad Autónoma de Nuevo León. [Muscular resistance exercise in physical functionality of older adults. Unpublished doctoral dissertation, Autonomous University of Nuevo Leon, School of Nursing, Monterrey, Mexico].

Derogatis, L. (1985). The psychosocial adjustment to illness scale. *Journal of Psychosomatic Research, 1*(30), 77–91.

Esquivel-Rodríguez & García Campos. (2007). Nivel de adaptación en el modo fisiológico: actividad y descanso del adulto mayor con hipertensión arterial. [Adaptation level to the physiological mode: activity and rest of the elderly with hypertension.] *Desarrollo Científico de Enfermería, 15*(6), 245–249.

Fawcett, J. (1999). *The relationship of theory and research* (3rd ed.). Philadelphia PA: Davis.

Gallegos, E. C., Cárdenas, V. M., & Salas, M. T. (1999). Capacidades de autocuidado del adulto con diabetes tipo 2. [Self-care abilities of adults with type 2 diabetes]. *Investigación y Educación en Enfermería, 8*(2), 23–33.

Gallegos, E. C., Ovalle-Berúmen, J. F., & Gómez-Meza, M. V. (2006). Metabolic control of adults with type 2 diabetes mellitus through education and counseling. *Journal of Nursing Scholarship, 38*(4), 344–351.

García-Valenzuela, M. L. R., Cuevas-Cansino, J. J., & Tinoco-López, G. (2004). Nivel de adaptación de los pacientes oncológicos a la quimioterapia ambulatoria. [Adaptation level of cancer patients to outpatient chemotherapy]. *Desde la Ciencias de la Salud, 1*, 2–5.

Gordon Gordon, M. (1987). *Manual of nursing diagnosis 1984–1985: including all diagnostic categories accepted by the North American Nursing Diagnosis Association.* NY: McGraw-Hill.

Gutierrez-López, C.,Veloza-Gómez, M. M., Moreno-Ferguson, M. E., Durán de Villalobos, M. M., López de Mesa, C., & Crespo, O. (2007). Validez y confiabilidad de la versión en español del instrumento "Escala de medición del proceso de afrontamiento y adaptación" de Callista Roy. [Validity and reliability of the Spañish version of the instrument "Coping process and adaptation scale" of Callista Roy.] *Aquichán, 7*(1), 54–63.

Gutiérrez-Valverde, J. M. (2010). Riesgo de desarrollar diabetes tipo 2: Interacción genmedio ambiente. Tesis de Doctoral no publicada, Universidad Autónoma de Nuevo León-Facultad de Enfermería. [Risk of developing type 2 diabetes: Gene-environment interaction. Unpublished dissertation, Autonomous University of Nuevo Leon, School of Nursing, Monterrey, Mexico].

Henderson, V. (1978). *Principles and practice of nursing.* London: Collier Mcmillan.

Hernandez, L., & Blazer, D. G. (eds) (2006). *Genes, behavior and the social environment. Moving beyond the nature/nurture debate.* Washington, D. C. National Academic Press.

Hernández-Méndez, E. I., Martínez-González, M. D., & Landeros-Olvera, E. (2009). Capacidades de autocuidado en adultos con hipertensión arterial y adultos sanos. [Self-care abilities in adults with hypertension and healthy adults]. *Desarrollo Científico de Enfermería, 17*(5), 207–211.

Hospital Ángeles Pedregal (n. d.). *Modelo de Gestión del Cuidado de Enfermería [Management model of nursing care].* Retrieved from http://www.up.edu.mx/files_uploads/15577_modelo.pdf

Kantun-Marín, M. A. J. (2012). Estímulos focales y contextuales en respuestas adaptativas para el envejecimiento exitoso en adultos mayores. Tesis doctoral inédita, Universidad Autónoma de Nuevo León, Monterrey, México. [Focal and contextual stimuli in adaptive responses to successful aging in older adults. Unpublished doctoral dissertation, Autonomous University of Nuevo Leon, School of Nursing, Monterrey, Mexico].

King, I. M. (1981). *A theory for nursing systems, concepts and process.* Albany: Delmar Thomson Learning.

Landeros, E. A., & Gallegos-Cabriales, E. C. (2005). Capacidades de autocuidado y percepción del estado de salud en adultos con y sin obesidad. [Self-care abilities and perceived health status in adults with or without obesity]. *Revista Mexicana de Enfermería Cardiológica, 13*, 20–24.

Landeros-Olvera, E. A. (2010). Intervención de ejercicio con base en el modelo de Roy en mujeres con sobrepeso y obesidad: Efectos fisiológicos y de auto concepto. Tesis doctoral inédita, Universidad Autónoma de Nuevo León, Monterrey, México. [Exercise intervention based on Roy's model in overweight and obese women: Physiological and self-concept effects. Unpublished doctoral dissertation, Autonomous University of Nuevo Leon, School of Nursing, Monterrey, Mexico].

Lazcano-Ortíz, M., & Salazar-González, B. C. (2008). Validación del instrumento: afrontamiento y proceso de adaptación de Roy en pacientes con diabetes mellitus tipo 2. [Instrument validation: Coping and Roy's adaptation processes in patients with type 2 diabetes mellitus.]. *Aquichán, 8*(1), 116–125.

Lazcano-Ortíz, M., & Salazar-González, B. C. (2009). Adaptación en pacientes con diabetes mellitus tipo 2, según Modelo de Roy. [Adaptation in patients with type 2 diabetes mellitus, according to Roy's model]. *Aquichán, 9*(3), 236–245.

Marriner-Tomey, A., & Alligood, M. R. (2008). Modelos y teorías en enfermería. [Nursing theorists and their work]. (6th ed.). Barcelona: Elsevier.

Maya-Morales, A., & Fonseca-Castaño, M. (2008). El Apoyo Familiar en la Adaptación y Autocuidado del Paciente con Diabetes Mellitus tipo 2. [Family support in adaptation and self-care of patients with type 2 diabetes mellitus]. *Desarrollo Científico de Enfermería, 16*(1), 15–18.

Medellín-Vélez, B. (2007). Desarrollo de capacidades de auto-cuidado en personas con diabetes mellitus tipo 2 [Development of self-care agency in individuals with type 2 diabetes mellitus]. *Revista de Enfermería del Instituto Mexicano del Seguro Social, 15*(2), 91–98.

Meleis, A. I. (2012). *Theoretical nursing: Development & progress* (5th ed.). Philadelphia: Wolters Kluwer.

Méndez-Salazar, V., Becerril-Estrada, V., Morales-Pilar, M., & Pérez-Ilagor, V. M. (2010). Autocuidado de las adultas mayores con diabetes mellitus inscritas en el progama de enfermedades crónicas de Temoaya México [Self-care of older adults with diabetes mellitus enrolled in the chronic diseases program of Temoaya Mexico]. *Ciencias y Enfermería, 16*(3), 103–109.

Muñoz-Canché, K. A. (2001) Ejercicio de resistencia muscular en adultos con diabetes mellitus tipo 2. Tesis de maestria no publicada. [Endurance training in adults with diabetes mellitus type 2. Master Thesis]. Universidad Autónoma de Nuevo León.

NANDA International (2011). *Nursing diagnoses 2012–2014. Definitions and classifications.* UK: Whiley Blackwell.

Neuman, B., & Fawcett, J. (2011). *The Neuman systems model.* Fifth ed. USA: Parson.

Orem, D. E. (2001). *Nursing concepts of practice,* 6th ed. St L ouis: Mossby.

Pender, N. J., Murdaugh C. L., & Parsons, M. A. (2002). The health promotion model. In N. J. Pender, C. L. Murdaugh, M. A. Parsons (eds.). In *Health promotion in nursing practice.* (4th ed.). Englewood Cliffs: Prentice Hall.

Rosales-Barrera, S., & Reyes-Gómez, E. (2004). *Fundamentos de Enfermería. México: Manual Moderno* [*Fundamentals of nursing.* Mexico: Modern Manual].

Roy, C., & Andrews, H. E. (1991). Essentials of the Roy adaptation model. In C. Roy, H. E. Andrews (eds.). In *The Roy adaptation model: The definitive statement.* Norwalk: Appleton & Lange.

Roy, C., & Andrews, H. E. (1999). Essentials of the Roy adaptation model. In C. Roy, H. E. Andrews (eds.). In *The Roy adaptation model.* Stamford: Appleton & Lange.

Roy, C. (2009). Elements of the Roy adaptation model. In *The Roy Adaptation Model.* (3rd ed.). Upper Saddle River, New Jersey: Pearson.

Sánchez-Meza, N. H. (2012). Estado de salud capacidades y cuidado dependiente del cuidador del adulto con T2DM. Tesis de MCE no publicada, Universidad Autónoma de Nuevo León-Facultad de Enfermería. [Health status abilities and dependent care of the caregiver for adults with T2DM. Unpublished thesis, Autonomous University of Nuevo Leon, School of Nursing, Monterrey, Mexico].

Secretaría de Salud (SSA), Subsecretaría de Integración y Desarrollo del Sector Salud, & Dirección General de Calidad y Educación en Salud (2011). *Lineamiento General Para la Elaboración de Planes de Cuidados de Enfermería.* [Secretariat of Health, Undersecretariat for Integration and Development of the Healthcare Sector & Directorate General of Quality and Health Education (2011). *General guideline for development of nursing care plans*]. Retrieved from http://www.salud.gob.mx/unidades/cie/cms_cpe/

Secretaría de Salud (SSA), Subsecretaría de Integración y Desarrollo del Sector Salud, & Dirección General de Calidad y Educación en Salud (2012). *Primer Catálogo Nacional de Planes de Cuidados de Enfermería.* [Secretariat of Health, Undersecretariat for Integration and Development of the Healthcare Sector & Directorate General of Quality and

Health Education (2012*). First national catalogue of nursing care plans].* Retrieved from http://www.salud.gob.mx/unidades/cie/cms_cpe/

Secretaría de Salud (SSA), Subsecretaría de Integración y Desarrollo del Sector Salud, & Dirección General de Calidad y Educación en Salud (2013). *Primer Catálogo Nacional de Planes de Cuidados de Enfermería.* [Secretariat of Health, Under Secretariat for Integration and Development of the Healthcare Sector & Directorate General of Quality and Health Education (2013). *Second national catalogue of nursing care plans].* Retrieved from http://www.salud.gob.mx/unidades/cie/cms_cpe/

Vicente-Ruiz, M. A. (2006). Capacidades y autocuidado en adolescentes en riesgo de DT2: Efecto de una intervención de ejercicio y orientación alimentaria. Tesis de DCE no publicada, Universidad Autónoma de Nuevo León-Facultad de Enfermería. [Skills and self-care in adolescents at risk for T2DM: Effect of an exercise intervention and dietary guidance. Unpublished thesis, Autonomous University of Nuevo Leon, School of Nursing].

Villarreal-Reyna, M. A. (2006). Programa psicoeducativo en familiares cuidadores de personas con la enfermedad de Alzheimer. Tesis doctoral inédita, Universidad Autónoma de Nuevo León. [Psychoeducational program for family caregivers of people with Alzheimer's disease. Unpublished doctoral dissertation, Autonomous University of Nuevo Leon, School of Nursing, Monterrey, Mexico].

Watson, J. (2011). *Nursing the philosophy and science of caring.* Revised edition. University Press of Colorado.

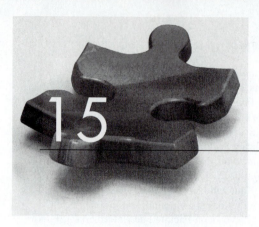

Thailand: Nursing Theory and Theory-Based Education, Practice, and Research

Natawon Suwonnaroop, Wanpen Piyopasakul, and Rungnapa Panitrat

INTRODUCTION

Thailand, known in history as Siam, is a unique country in Southeast Asia with a combination of traditional beliefs and modern practices. In relation to nursing and health care practices, Thailand has long employed local wisdom and traditional medicine to manage health issues (Ministry of Public Health, 2007). Like many other countries around the world, modernization has gradually made its way to the Thai nation to improve the quality of life of its people. Nursing education in Thailand has also changed from a traditional approach to one in which many modern nursing and midwifery programs are now available in university nursing schools.

From 1896 onwards, modern nursing has evolved throughout the country. This evolution took place simultaneously with the establishment of the first hospital in Thailand, namely "Siriraj Hospital." The hospital, located in Bangkok, was established in 1888 to provide health care services for Thai patients. However, many Thais were reluctant to come to the hospital because they were not familiar with modern medicine and preferred home remedies. Later, when satisfaction with hospital care gradually increased among the public, more Thai people took advantage of the hospital

198

services offered (Thaweeboon, Peachpansri, Pochanapan, Senachack, & Pinyopasakul, 2011).

BACKGROUND: DEVELOPMENT OF NURSING IN THAILAND

For the past century, Thailand has experienced many economic and political issues. Despite this, the growth and development of Thai nursing education has continued. Currently, Thailand has more than 60 university nursing schools offering a wide range of nursing programs for both Thai and international students. These programs range from bachelor's and master's degree programs to doctoral studies (Thailand Nursing and Midwifery Council, 2015). In addition, some nursing programs need to be specifically developed in order to meet the demands of health care issues in the country. For example, in 2002 the Thailand Nursing and Midwifery Council (TNMC) approved a 4-month training curriculum for general nurse practitioners to serve the demands of government policy in providing nurse practitioners in all health-promoting hospitals at subdistrict levels within 10 years. At the same time, many nursing educational institutes developed a master's program for advanced practice nurses (APNs) based on the U.S. model within six clinical nursing specialists (surgical/medical, pediatrics, maternal/newborn, mental health/psychiatric, community health, and gerontological nursing) as well as family/community nurse practitioners. Nurses are expected to be more knowledgeable than previously and skillful in providing expert nursing care based on theory and evidence-based practice to promote healthy behaviors and reduce health threats across the care delivery continuum. Certainly, a proliferation of nursing schools and advanced nursing courses in the Thai nation reflect the remarkable progress of Thai nursing over time. Since 1977, nursing theories have gradually emerged and have become a path to progress in the Thai nursing profession.

EVOLUTION OF NURSING EDUCATION IN THAILAND

The first Thai nursing school, which now is the Faculty of Nursing, Mahidol University, was founded under the patronage of Her Majesty Queen Sripatcharintra on January 12, 1896. Initially, Thai nursing education evolved from a hospital-based program, an apprentice-training model taught by male physicians. The nursing school focused largely on midwifery and nursing curriculum including principles of sanitary practice, management of communicable diseases, medication administration, mental health support, and childrearing. During 1926–1935, Thailand engaged in many exchanges and agreements with Western countries; thus, the evolution of Thai nursing education took place under the influences of Western missionary nurses and doctors (Bhongbhiphat, Reynolds, & Polpatpichar, 1983).

A program of nursing education was fully developed when His Royal Highness Prince Mahidol of Songkla, widely known as the "Father of Modern Medicine and Public Health" in Thailand, brought two U.S. nurse educators to Bangkok in 1926 with support from the Rockefeller Foundation to revise the existing programs. Since then, more structural changes in nursing education have occurred, such as introducing public health courses into the nursing curriculum. In 1956, a four-year program leading to a degree of bachelor of science in nursing was established as the first baccalaureate nursing program in the country. The establishment of the baccalaureate nursing program is recognized as the transition of professional nursing from hospital-based training to a university education (Thaweeboon, Peachpansri, Pochanapan, Senachack, & Pinyopasakul, 2011). However, the curriculum had no nursing theories until the first master of nursing science program was introduced in 1977 at the Faculty of Nursing, Mahidol University. The standards of nursing education in Thailand have been identified as contributing to the country's growth and development.

Theories Used in Nursing In Thailand

In 1977, Tassana Boontong, a Thai nurse educator and leader, introduced the first nursing theories in Thailand as subjects for the master's of nursing science program. Subsequently, other nursing theories have been taught in nursing schools in Thailand and are widely recognized throughout the country. In 1987, nursing theory was first included as a core subject in the baccalaureate nursing program at the Faculty of Nursing, Mahidol University and was later introduced to other Thai nursing schools. When a doctorate of nursing science program was initiated in 1989 at the Faculty of Nursing, Mahidol University, the subject of nursing theory development was integrated as a core subject in the curriculum (Faculty of Nursing, Mahidol University, 1996). Thus, nursing theories have been included in Thai nursing education for more than 30 years and continue to contribute to the growth and development of nursing in the country.

HEALTH CARE DELIVERY SYSTEMS IN THAILAND

From past to present, the nursing profession has been one of the key agents contributing to the successful development of Thailand's health care delivery system. This system has evolved from preventive services to controlling communicable diseases and to modern medical care. The baccalaureate-prepared nurse is the minimum credential for practicing as a professional nurse in the health care services system; master's and doctoral nursing graduates take part in the development of nurses' roles and improvement of the nursing and health care services.

Prior to 1978, self-reliance was central to the health care system in Thai society. This means that Thai people had learned to care for themselves or others, sometimes with the assistance of folk or lay people, or local wisdom from their communities (Ministry of Public Health, 2007) and relied heavily on this type of care. There were no hospitals in the country before the 19th century.

Modern health care came to Thailand in the late 17th century when missionaries brought Western medical science with them. King Chulalongkorn founded the first general hospital, Siriraj Hospital, in 1886 in Bangkok and became a more accepted and medical source in many regions. To date, the health care system in Thailand has evolved with many changes and developments in its policies and organizations. Nevertheless, self-reliance has remained an important aspect of the Thai health care system to foster self care among the Thai population (Ministry of Public Health, 2007).

Organization of Thai Health Care System

The health care system in Thailand is mainly organized and delivered by the public sector. The Ministry of Public Health (MoPH) is the major institution responsible for providing public health and medical services nationwide through a three-tiered delivery system: (a) primary care (small community hospitals with 10 beds and health centers at the subdistrict level), (b) secondary care (community hospitals at district level with 30–150 beds), and (c) tertiary care (provincial and regional hospitals with 200–1,000 beds) (Nitayarumpong & Pannarumothai, 1997; Wibulpolprasert, 2008). Private hospitals and clinics also provide health and medical services throughout the country; they are widespread in urban areas. People who live in remote or rural areas often have limited access to health care services, although they receive some help from primary health care personnel. In hospitals, nurses primarily practice using the medical disease-oriented model because of its hospital-based origin. Public health nurses, however, usually perform their roles in both in-service and outreach activities for health promotion, prevention, and control of diseases and health hazards for individuals, families, and communities.

Health Care Reform

In 1977, the Thai government implemented primary health care (PHC) as the foundation of health care delivery to improve it on the basis of health care needs; it sought to approach a *health for all* policy. Under PHC, nurses and public health staff have a significant role in training "grass-roots" village health volunteers in Thailand. These volunteers focus on health education, family planning, basic treatment, maternal and child health care, and prevention of local diseases. Many innovative health activities, such as community organization, community self-financing and management, health system restructure, and multisectoral coordination, were established in local communities to strengthen community self-reliance and improve people's quality of life (Nitayarumpong, 1990).

In 2000, Thailand experienced a health care reform as the result of the country's economic crisis. The government was forced to cope with socio-economic changes driven by globalization that widely led to unhealthy lifestyles of the Thai people. In response to the health for all policy, the five strategies of the Ottawa Charter for Health Promotion of the World Health Organization (WHO, 1986) have been adapted into a more proactive approach for disease prevention and health promotion in hospitals and in the community, such as home-based care and the establishment of elderly clubs and child care centers. Prevention of chronic disease and the promotion of healthy lifestyles were addressed as one of major development goals in the Ninth National Health Development Plan under the Ninth Economic and Social Development Plan (2002–2006). The Ninth National Health Development Plan (Bureau of Policy and Strategy, Ministry of Public Health, 2005) shifted the focus of health care from an economic-based plan to a human-centered development approach to ensure sustainable and balanced development for living together peacefully with nature and the environment (Bureau of Policy and Strategy, Ministry of Public Health, 2012). His Majesty the King's philosophy of *sufficiency economy* (SE) has been applied as the guiding framework for development of people's health and the restructuring of the health system into the Ninth National Health Plan. The SE philosophy emphasizes appropriate conduct and way of life that incorporates three aspects: moderation (not too little, not too much), reasonableness (being aware of what one is doing and why), and self-immunity (inner resilience to deal with unexpected shocks) (United Nations Development Programme, 2007). The development of these three concepts requires the application of accurate knowledge and ethics in the forms of care and giving, mutual assistance, and collaboration to create sustainable and appropriate health care services.

In 2001, a universal health coverage scheme (UCS) was launched to cover all Thai people who were not covered by other health protection plans. UCS provided equitable access to comprehensive health care services (Buasai, Kanchanachitra, & Siwaraksa, 2007). Since then, UCS has covered about 75% of the country's population, and the civil servant medical benefit scheme (SMBS) and social security scheme (SSS) together cover approximately 22%. The UCS study project recommended that delivery should be shifted to focus on the primary care system as a gatekeeper to provide prevention, health risk appraisal, health promotion, particularly behavior modification, and reconstruction more than curative service (Chunharas, 2005). The community medical center and subdistrict health-promoting hospital (newly named *health center*) serve as the primary care facilities. Moreover, the hospital health-promoting master plan, which integrates health promotion in hospital services and is more health oriented than curative oriented, has been developed and implemented in MoPH hospitals. The goals of this plan are to enhance people's integrity and give them the ability to control their own health and illness as well as to empower hospital staff to become role models in providing supportive physical, social, and spiritual environments (Auamkul & Kanshana, 2003).

Meanwhile, MoPH required a reduction in health care costs that could be achieved by strengthening ambulatory or home health services. Integrated health services, which involve health care institutions, families, and community support systems, have become a focus of the service delivery reform to manage both patient care and budget concerns effectively. These initiatives were crucial to Thailand's efforts to progress toward almost all health-related millennium development goals. The decrease in infant and maternal mortality rates and the increase of life expectancy at birth demonstrate the achievement of these goals (Bureau of Policy and Strategy, Ministry of Public Health, 2012). To date, the SE philosophy has been applied to the nursing profession and has become a key element in the achievement of excellence in the nursing profession in Thailand.

Essentially, the Ninth National Health Development Plan in Thailand (Bureau of Policy and Strategy, Ministry of Public Health, 2005) increasingly adopts the King Bhumibol's philosophy of SE, which emphasizes a human-centered development approach, multisectoral cooperation, and active participation from the public in the decision-making process (Bureau of Policy and Strategy, 2011). Preventive measures and health promotion are addressed in the program management to reduce health risk problems, to build capacity of self care for individuals, families, and communities, and to develop immunity against external threats. In response to this need, nurses and APNs in all levels of the health service system, including primary care and hospital settings, are recognized for their significant role in and contribution to leading change and improving client and community health outcomes (Pender, Murdaugh, & Parsons, 2011; Milstead, 2013). The development of the professional competency and leadership attributes are deemed necessary if the country wishes to remodel nursing education. There is a global health agenda of epidemiological transition and workforce shortages in nursing and health care (Frenk et al., 2010).

Thai Nursing Education Redesign

As a result of health care reforms and the shift in emphasis from acute illnesses to noncommunicable diseases and an increase in the higher education of nursing in Thailand, all nursing schools redesigned their nursing curricula and utilized health promotion as a framework for nursing education and theory. In the undergraduate as well as postgraduate programs, health promotion has been emphasized to prepare nurses regarding the essential knowledge of human behavior, factors contributing to health, as well as the principles and strategic approaches to health promotion. Teaching and learning activities in each nursing school vary according to the major concepts or theories being taught. Certainly, nurse educators are challenged to design teaching and learning models that stimulate students' inquiry-based learning and enhance skills for performing health promotion activities and projects in various groups of population, such as risk groups and healthy people. (Suwonnaroop, 2011; Phutthikamin, 2011). The Health Promotion Nursing Network (HPNN) in Thailand published a handbook (Sritanyarat, Sutra, Aroonsang, & Lertrat, 2012) for health promotion in the bachelor of nursing curriculum as a guide for nursing educators. It was distributed to all academic nursing institutes. Pender's health promotion model (Pender, 1996), health belief model (Rosenstock, 1974), and the empowerment concept (WHO, 2006) have been introduced into this teaching handbook.

Health Promotion Theory Course

To evaluate the outcome after use of health promotion theory, Tassniyom (2011) conducted a health promotion course for bachelor of science students, which based empowerment as one of the core concepts of health promotion. Students were divided into groups of 20; each student was required to evaluate his or her health condition, identify areas of behavior adjustment, use evidence-based research for planning and implementing health behavior changes, and evaluate the outcomes of these activities. Students were encouraged to report their ideas to the nursing instructor through a mentor of each group. This learning method helped the students to comprehend their own strengths and weakness through self-performed health care, self-responsibility, self-esteem, pride, problem-solving skills, and self-criticism.

Risk Factors from Noncommunicable Diseases

Thailand, like other Asian and Western countries, is facing high mortality and morbidity rates from noncommunicable diseases (NCDs) and an increase in the aging population. For example, Suwanwela (2014) reported that the prevalence of cerebrovascular diseases in Thai people has been increasing with the mean age of 65 years old, leading to greater mortality and long term disability. Health is now heavily influenced by a broad range of multiple factors of health and social determinants that are driven by current globalization, capitalist economy, and communication technology (Bureau of Policy and Strategy, Ministry of Public Health, 2011). Four main behavioral risk factors are tobacco use, harmful use of alcohol, insufficient physical activity, and unhealthy diet. As revealed in its 2008–2013 action plan, WHO (2008) developed a global strategy for preventing and controlling NCDs to provide international member communities with a road map and policy options to establish and strengthen initiatives for surveillance, prevention, and management of NCDs. Thailand's healthy lifestyle strategic plan (2011–2020) was also developed in response to the need to address preventable lifestyle diseases.

In addition to NCDs, vehicle accident is another health-related problem in Thailand. The United Nations (2013) ranks Thailand as the third in the list of countries having highest road traffic deaths worldwide with 38.1 road fatalities per 100,000 inhabitants per year in 2010. Driving over the speed limit and drunk driving are major causes of accidents (Ponboon, Islam, Boontob, Kanitpong, & Tanaboriboon, 2010). The context of health issues is now more complex and dynamic than previously. Consequently, diverse theories are needed in order to understand and improve health behaviors. Western theories concerned with human behaviors and the influences of the environment were used as conceptual frameworks in nursing research by the year 2000.

RESEARCH ON TOPICS RELATED TO NURSING IN THAILAND

The greater complexity of health issues in Thai society has an impact on the advancement of nursing practice. Wongkpratoom, Srisuphan, Senaratana, Nantachaipan, and Sritanyarat (2010) explored the development of APNs' role in Thailand using both quantitative and qualitative approaches. They collected the quantitative data regarding the APN role performance from 154 APNs who had been certified between 2003 and 2005 and worked in hospitals and primary care settings. The study's results showed that the APN's role performance was high in the roles of direct clinical care, educator, consultant, administrator, and researcher. They also conducted an in-depth interview with 13 APNs working in clinical settings located in various regions of Thailand to understand the APN's role development. The findings revealed three stages of APN's role development: advanced beginner, competent practitioner, and expert. The major factors for facilitating APN role development were (a) organization (health care system and organizational policies), (b) human (quality of administrator and well-functioning multidisciplinary teams), and (c) resources (financial assistance). Previously, there were two studies using nursing experts to examine the conceptual structure of care competencies (Nontapet, Isaramalai, Petpichatchain, & Brook, 2008; Ruksaphram, Isaramalai, & Bunyasopun, 2014). Nontapet and collegues (Nontapet, Isaramalai, Petpichatchain, & Brook, 2008) examined the primary care competency among primary care nurses and found four major domains of the competency components: interpersonal relationship, care management, integrated health care service, and professional accountability, whereas Ruksaphram, Isaramalai, and Bunyasopun (2014) conducted a study with primary care providers, including public health staff, doctors, and nurses, and found four domains of chronic care competency: behavior risk management, symptom management, treatment prescription, and health coaching. These two studies have suggested that nurses need to improve their competencies to manage with complex health issues, and advanced nursing should be integrated into the nursing curriculum for graduate nurses in primary care and other clinical settings.

In graduate programs, health promotion is one of the research areas in both the master's and doctoral programs. The health promotion model (HPM) developed by Pender (1987; 1996) is one of the most popular conceptual frameworks used for nursing research. From 1998 to 2001, 47 theses, dissertations, or published manuscripts used HPM as a guiding research conceptual framework (Tilokskulchai, Sitthimongkol, Prasopkitikun, & Klainin, 2004). Most of these studies sought to determine personal characteristics and behavior-specific cognition in predicting overall health-promoting behaviors and risk behaviors. Forty-five percent of these studies selected adults with chronic illnesses as the population of interest. For example, Jianvitayakij, Panpakdee, Malathum, Duffy, and Viwatwongkasem (2014) conducted a descriptive correlational study to determine the predictive factors of smoking cessation in a sample of 280 Thai male smokers with hypertension using the 1996 HPM version. Individual characteristics (age, education, level of nicotine independence, concern about the harm of smoking) and behavior-specific cognition (perceived benefits, perceived barriers, perceived self-efficacy, and social support for smoking cessation) were selected to predict the smoking cessation behavior. The findings showed that perceived self-efficacy of smoking cessation and concern about the harm of smoking accounted for 68% of the variance in smoking cessation behavior. These studies could be used to inform other nursing interventions to improve the outcomes of health-promoting behaviors among Thai people.

Medicine and nursing education and practice in Thailand have evolved since the late 1800s (Kunaviktikul, 2006), but nursing research did not gain local and national attention until 1970 when the first two-year master's program in nursing was offered and the doctoral program in public health nursing followed in 1985. Subsequently, nursing research emerged in the form of master's theses or doctoral dissertations, which are required to fulfill the degree. For example, the findings from a meta-analysis study entitled *"Factors related to health promoting behaviors among older adults: A meta-analysis"* revealed that 77% of these studies were master's degree theses (Thanakwang, Kespichayawattana, & Jittapanya, 2010). Another example is the study entitled *"A survey of nursing research related to diabetic patients in Thailand,"* which demonstrated that most nursing research studies in Thailand were from master's theses and doctoral dissertations (Menetthip, 1997).

In Thailand, Western nursing theories have been used as conceptual frameworks for conducting nursing research and were primarily used to guide descriptive, predictive, and intervention research. Those theories included Orem's (1991) self-care, Roy's (2009) adaptation, and Pender's (1996) health promotion models. As revealed in the study of Kattika, Jiraporn, Chanokporn (2010), 75% of the health promotion research using Pender's health promotion model or Orem's self-care model was utilized among different groups in studies of various populations and settings. Interestingly, after 2000, nursing theories have not been used exclusively, and theories from related disciplines such as psychology, social work, and environmental science have been increasingly used. These theories include social cognition theories, such as Bandura's (1997) self-efficacy or Lazarus and Folkman's (1984) stress and coping. For example, a study on Thai adolescent suicide risk behavior, whose goal was to test a model of negative life events, rumination, emotional distress, resilience, and social support, used a cognitive theory instead of a nursing theory to explain the findings (Thanoi, Phancharoenworakul, Thompson, Panitrat, & Nityasuddh, 2010).

A critical analysis of the use of nursing theories in Thailand from 2000 to 2010 demonstrated that the country faced a rapidly changing environment that significantly influenced health and health care delivery systems. In the 2000, which is a starting point of the economic crisis, health problems in Thailand dramatically changed from infectious diseases to NCDs, including heart disease, hypertension, diabetes mellitus, renal failure, and stroke. These changes resulted from a rapidly evolving environment that significantly affected the country. The NCDs have emerged as a result of social and environmental changes in the country, causing changes in daily lifestyles that affect individual behavior and the ecology. Consequently, diverse theories are needed in order to understand and improve health behaviors. Western theories concerned with human behaviors and the influences of the environment were used as conceptual frameworks in nursing research by the year 2000.

Furthermore, from 2001–2005, the Ninth National Health Plan highlighted two areas. First, its planning process shifted from "for the people, by the government" to "people's participation" (National Economic and Social Development Board Office of the Prime Minister, 2011). This agenda influenced research methodology, with many research studies focusing more on the participation of all stakeholders and sustainability of the health care system that leads to optimal health and health care outcomes. Conceptual frameworks have then shifted from Western philosophies to a local tailor-made perspective, such as the SE philosophy established by King Bhumibol Adulyadej. Meanwhile, the Healthcare Accreditation Institute was established to scrutinize and certify health care settings around Thailand. Since 2000, Thai health care services have been reorganized to ensure the quality of care. In response to need for evidence-based practices, health care practitioners called for a research agenda that sought to improve quality of nursing and health care. Therefore, many research studies, especially master's theses, were conducted on this issue, and these evidence-based practices were used as important tools to evaluate nursing actions.

Although the conduct of research has been well developed, the National Research Council of Thailand (NRCT) noted the lack of research utilization among Thai health care professionals. The Health Systems Research Institute and NRCT therefore launched the project called "*Ghan Wijai Chai Jing–Jak Hing sue Hang*" (in Thai), or "*Research utilization–From shelf to department store*" in 2005 (Health Systems Research Institute, 2014). Its objective is to stimulate research utilization in routine practices in clinical and community settings. Consequently, the project called "*from routine to research (R2R)*" was launched to improve the quality of care that aimed to integrate life and work with practical research. Since then, more nursing research has been produced by Thai nurses in health care settings and in communities.

Although nursing intervention evaluation research is now in demand and is being undertaken, there has been less emphasis on health system research. In this time of transition of economic, social, and environmental changes in Thailand, it is necessary to conduct health system research that results from the (a) complexity of health problems and (b) emphasis of the Tenth National Health Plan (reinforcing the structure, mechanisms, and processes of the administration). Previous research studies in Thai nursing appear to have focused more on humans, health, and nursing with a narrow focus on other issues, such as environment. The environmental issue is less well defined and focuses mainly on small settings (e.g., family or a community).

Overall, the question of what Thai nursing research should focus on with high expectation for effectiveness and limited resources in the country's rapid social change remains unanswered. A few suggestions for future nursing research are offered.

> First, research should emphasize issues regarding the promotion of healthy behaviors in healthy, at risk, and sick people.

> Second, more research should focus on creating a safe environment not only in clinical settings but also in the realms of social, physical, psychological, and environmental safety.

> Third, more research on the effectiveness of health care services or nursing interventions is needed, especially for people with chronic illness and for elders, who are the largest population of care recipients.

> Finally, to enhance the outcomes of health care and nursing services, the use of a single theory may not be sufficient for both nursing education and nursing research in Thailand. Because the country has proposed a shared vision of "a happy society with equality, fairness and resilience" (National Economic and Social Development Board Office of the Prime Minister, 2011), the SE philosophy is now widely integrated with health care policy and practices to achieve balanced and sustainable development. Concerns with the country's specific context is a significant key to address the difficulties or hindrances to successfully protecting and promoting people's health.

CONCLUSION

This chapter describes nursing theory and theory-based education, practice, and research in Thailand. The chapter discussed the emergence of nursing theory from a Western context in the country for more than three decades. It also explained some nursing theories and how they were introduced and utilized. Currently, changes are occurring in Thai health care systems, policies, and service deliveries. Clearly, the health care environment, characteristics of patients and illnesses, and economic issues create a high demand for nurses to work in what is now a more complex environment. Therefore, the use of nursing theory must be congruent with it. Theory should be used in an integrative way that is context based and culturally appropriate to best guide nursing education, practice, and research in the country.

REFERENCES

Auamkul, N., & Kanshana, S. (2003). *Development of health promoting hospital in Thailand*. Retrieved 12 March 2015 from http://unpan1.un.org/intradoc/groups/public/documents/apcity/unpan009705.pdf

Bandura, A. (1997). *Self-efficacy: The exercise of control*. New York: W. H. Freeman.

Bhongbhiphat, V., Reynolds, B., & Polpatpichar, S. (1983). *The eagle and the elephant: 150 years of Thai-American relations*. Bangkok: United Production.

Buasai S. I., Kanchanachitra C, & Siwaraksa P. (2007). The way forward: Experiences of health promotion development in Thailand. *Promotion and Education, 14*(4), 250–253.

Bureau of Policy and Strategy, Ministry of Public Health. (2005). *Thai public health (2001–2004)*. Nonthaburi, Thailand: Ministry of Public Health.

Bureau of Policy and Strategy, Ministry of Public Health. (2011). *Thailand Healthy Lifestyle Strategic Plan (2011–2020)*. Nonthaburi, Thailand: Ministry of Public Health.

Bureau of Policy and Strategy, Ministry of Public Health. (2012). *The 11th Health National Development Plan under the National Economic and Social Development Plan B.E 2555–2559 (A.D. 2012–2016)*. Bangkok: War Veterans Organization Office of Printing Mill.

Chunharas, S. (2005). *Health service delivery system vs. health infrastructure systems: Problems and recommendation for development*. Nonthaburi, Thailand: Health System Research Institute.

Faculty of Nursing, Mahidol University. (1996). *A hundred years school of nursing, midwifery, and public health at Siriraj*. Bangkok: Author.

Frenk, J., Chen, L., Bhutta, Z. A., Cohen, J., Crisp, N., Evan, T., et al. (2010). Health professionals for a new century: Transforming education to strengthen health system in an interdependent world. *The Lancet, 376*(9756), 1923–1958.

Health Systems Research Institute. (2014). *Health Systems Research Institute co-operates with National Research Council of Thailand to foster staff for research development and integration to policy (in Thai)*. Retrieved 19 September 2014 from http://www.hsri.or.th/researcher/media/news/detail/5780.

Jianvitayakij, S., Panpakdee, O., Malathum, P., Duffy, S. A., & Viwatwongkasem C., (2014). Factors influencing smoking cessation behavior among Thai male smokers with hypertension. *Pacific Rim International of Nursing Research, 18*(2), 100–110.

Kattika, T., Jiraporn, K., & Chanokporn, J. (2010). Factors related to health promoting behaviors among older adults: A meta-analysis, *Journal of Nursing Science, 28*(3), 60–68.

Kunaviktikul, W. (2006). Nursing and nursing education in Thailand: The past, the present, and the future. *Nursing and Health Sciences, 8*, 199–200.

Lazarus, R. S., & Folkman, S. (1984). *Stress, appraisal, and coping*. New York: Springer.

Menetthip, S. (1997). *A survey of nursing research related diabetic patients in Thailand*. Unpublished master's thesis, Mahidol University, Bangkok.

Milstead, M. A. (2013). *Health policy and politics: A nurse's guide* (4th ed.). Burlington, MA: Jones & Bartlett Learning.

Ministry of Public Health. (2007). *Thailand health profile report 2004–2007*. Nonthaburi, Thailand: Author.

National Economic and Social Development Board Office of the Prime Minister. (2011). *The eleventh national economic and social development plan (2012–2016)*. Nonthaburi, Thailand: Ministry of Public Health.

Nitayarumpong, S. (1990). Evolution of primary health care in Thailand: What policies worked? *Health Policy and Planning, 5*(3), 246–254.

Nitayarumpong, S., & Pannarunothai, S. (1997). Thailand at the crossroads: Challenges for health care reform. In S. Nitayarumpong (Ed.). *Health care reform at the frontier of research and policy decisions*. Nonthaburi, Thailand: Ministry of Public Health.

Nontapet, O., Isaramalai, S., Petpichatchain, W., & Brook, C. W. (2008). Conceptual structure of primary care competency for Thai primary care unit nurses. *Thai Journal of Nursing Research, 12*(3), 195–206.

Orem, D. E. (1991). *Nursing: Concepts of practice* (4th ed.). St. Louis, MO: Mosby.

Pender, N. J. (1987). *Health promotion in nursing practice* (2nd ed.). Norwalk, CT: Appleton & Lange.

Pender, N. J. (1996). *Health promotion in nursing practice* (3rd ed.). Norwalk, CT: Appleton & Lange.

Pender, N., Murdaugh, C., & Parsons, M. A. (2011). *Health promotion in nursing practice* (6th ed.). New York: Pearson Education.

Phutthikhamin, T. (2011). *The integration of health promotion concepts in the patients' assessment forms of clinical practice courses, bachelor of nursing science curriculum.* Khon Kaen: Faculty of Nursing, Khon Kaen University.

Ponboon, S., Islam, M. B., Boontob, N., Kanitpong, K., & Tanaboriboon, Y. (2010). Contributing factors of road crashes in Thailand: Evidences from the accident in-depth study. *Journal of the Eastern Asia Society for Transportation Studies, 8*(3), 1958–1970.

Rosenstock, I. M. (1974) Historical origins of the health belief model. *Health Education Monographs, 2*, 328–335.

Roy, C. (2009). *The Roy adaptation model* (3rd ed.). Upper Saddle River, NJ: Prentice Hall.

Ruksaphram, P., Isaramalai, S., & Bunyasopun, U. (2014). A conceptual structure of chronic care competency for Thai primary care providers. *Songklanagarind Journal of Nursing, 34*(1), 13–24.

Sritanyarat, W., Sutra, P., Aroonsang, P., & Lertrat, P. (2012). Compilation of research projects and innovations on health promotion: Health Promotion Nursing Network (HPNN) Phase II (2008–2011). *Thai Journal of Nursing Council, 27* (special issue), 114–212.

Suwanwela, N. C. (2014). Stroke epidemiology in Thailand. *Journal of Stroke, 16*(1), 1–7.

Suwonnaroop, N. (2011). Learning roadmap: A design of health promotion course. *Journal of Nursing Science, 29*(3), 103–107.

Tassniyom, N. (2011). Teaching health promotion based on the empowerment concept. *Thai Journal of Nursing Council, 26S* (special issue), 17–29.

Thailand Nursing and Midwifery Council. (2015). *Lists of nursing courses accredited by Thailand Nursing Council and Midwifery* (in Thai, update 13 February 2015). Retrieved 8 March 2015 from http://www.tnc.or.th/content/content-38.html

Thanakwang, K., Kespichayawattana, J., & Jittapanya, C. (2010). Factors related to health promoting behaviors among older adults: A meta-analysis. *Journal of Nursing Science, 28*(3), 60–68.

Thanoi, W., Phancharoenworakul, K., Thompson, E. A., Panitrat, R., & Nityasuddh D., (2010). Thai adolescent suicide risk behaviors: Testing a model of negative life events, rumination, emotional distress, resilience and social support. *Pacific Rim International Journal of Nursing Research, 14*(3), 187–202.

Thaweeboon, T., Peachpansri, S., Pochanapan, S., Senachack, S., & Pinyopasakul W., (2011). The history and development of the school of nursing, midwifery, and public health Siriraj from B.E. 2439 to 2514 (1896–1971). *Nursing and Health Sciences, 28*, 54–67.

Tilokskulchai, F., Sitthimongkol, Y., Prasopkittikul, T., & Klainin, P. (2004). Meta-analysis of health promotion research in Thailand. *Asian Journal of Nursing Studies, 7*(2), 18–32.

United Nations. (2013). *Statistical year book for Asia and the Pacific*. Retrieved 8 March 2015 from http://www.unescap.org/stat/data/syb2013/ESCAP-syb2013.pdf.

United Nations Development Programme. (2007). *Thailand human development report 2007: Sufficiency economy and human development*. Bangkok, Thailand: Author.

Wibulpolprasert, S. (2008). *Thailand health profile 2005–2007* (in Thai). Nonthaburi, Thailand: Ministry of Public Health. Retrieved 8 March 2015 from http://www.moph.go.th/ops/thp/thp/index.php?id=35&group_=01&page=view_doc

Wongkpratoom, S., Srisuphan, W., Senaratana, W., Nantachaipan, P., & Sritanyarat, W. (2010). Role development of advanced practice nurses in Thailand. *Pacific Rim International Journal of Nursing Research, 14*(2), 162–177.

World Health Organization. (1986). *The Ottawa Charter for health promotion*. Retrieved 8 March 2015 from http://www.who.int/healthpromotion/conferences/previous/ottawa/en/

World Health Organization. (2006). *What is the evidence on effectiveness of empowerment to improve health?* Retrieved 8 March 2015 from http://www.euro.who.int/__data/assets/pdf_file/0010/74656/E88086.pdf

World Health Organization. (2008). *2008–2013 Action plan for the global strategy for the prevention and control of noncommunicable diseases*. Retrieved 11 March 2015 from http://www.who.int/nmh/publications/ncd_action_plan_en.pdf

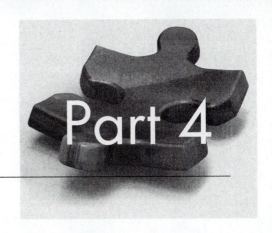

Part 4

Future Directions for Development of Nursing Theory, Research, and Professional Practice

CHAPTER OUTLINE

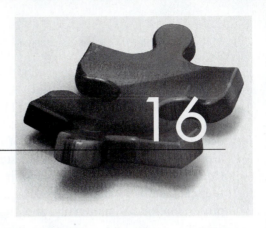

16

Nursing Knowledge Development and Professional Nursing Practice

Margaret Glembocki

PROFESSIONAL NURSING PRACTICE:

Professional nursing practice is the thoughtful representation of the complex and evolving knowledge that the discipline possesses. Each time a nurse uses the nursing process to make a clinical decision while providing individualized patient care or touches a suffering individual with intention, professional nursing practice is being demonstrated. It is not the task to be done but the thought and intention behind the action that creates professional nursing practice. The hands and thoughts of the professional nurses who are active in clinical practice embody the work of research and theory development within the discipline of nursing. Professional development of nursing practice formally began with the scientific writings of Florence Nightingale in 1860 when *Notes on Nursing: What It Is and What It Is Not* was published (Nightingale, 1860). She has been named the founder of modern nursing in response to this prolific work. Since this landmark publication, nursing has significantly developed and is practiced in every country throughout the world with approximately 14.5 million nurses globally (World Health Organization [WHO], 2011).

Understanding what represents a profession is essential to further development and implementation into clinical practice. Manthey (2002) has identified four characteristics that make a profession as opposed to an occupation. This is essential when examining professional development. The four characteristics are (1) identifiable body of knowledge that can best be transmitted in a formal educational program, (2) autonomy of decision making, (3) peer review of practice, and (4) identification with a professional organization as the standard setter and arbiter of practice (Manthey, 2). Currently, the discipline of nursing embodies each of these four characteristics and continues to support the further development of the profession locally, nationally, and globally.

Global Nursing Practice

The International Council of Nurses (ICN) is the global representation of professional nurses. It is a federation of more than 130 national associations representing nurses and the nursing profession globally. ICN (2014) has defined nursing as

> Nursing encompasses autonomous and collaborative care of individuals of all ages, families, groups and communities, sick or well and in all settings. Nursing includes the promotion of health, prevention of illness, and the care of ill, disabled and dying people. Advocacy, promotion of a safe environment, research, participation in shaping health policy and in patient and health systems management, and education are also key nursing roles.

The ICN first developed a worldwide code of ethics for nurses in 1953. It was revised in 2012 (ICN, 2012). The ICN code is a guide for action for all nurses based on social values and needs. It contains four principal elements: nurses and people, nurses and practice, nurses and the profession, and nurses and co-workers. The code presents detailed guidelines for practitioners, managers, educators, researchers, and national nurses associations for implementing the four elements.

1. Nurses and people
   • The nurse's primary professional responsibility is to people requiring nursing care.
   • In providing care, the nurse promotes an environment in which the human rights, values, customs and spiritual beliefs of the individual, family and community are respected.
   • The nurse ensures that the individual receives accurate, sufficient and timely information in a culturally appropriate manner on which to base consent for care and related treatment.
   • The nurse holds in confidence personal information and uses judgment in sharing this information.

- The nurse shares with society the responsibility for initiating and supporting action to meet the health and social needs of the public, in particular those of vulnerable populations.
- The nurse advocates for equity and social justice in resource allocation, access to health care, and other social and economic services.
- The nurse demonstrates professional values such as respectfulness, responsiveness, compassion, trustworthiness and integrity.

2. Nurses and practice
- The nurse carries personal responsibility and accountability for nursing practice, and for maintaining competence by continual learning.
- The nurse maintains a standard of personal health such that the ability to provide care is not compromised.
- The nurse uses judgment regarding individual competence when accepting and delegating responsibility.
- The nurse at all times maintains standards of personal conduct which reflect well on the profession and enhance its image and public confidence.
- The nurse, in providing care, ensures that use of technology and scientific advances are compatible with the safety, dignity, and rights of people.
- The nurse strives to foster and maintain a practice culture promoting ethical behavior and open dialogue.

3. Nurses and the profession
- The nurse assumes the major role in determining and implementing acceptable standards of clinical nursing practice, management, research, and education.
- The nurse is active in developing a core of research-based professional knowledge that supports evidence-based practice.
- The nurse is active in developing and sustaining a core of professional values.
- The nurse, acting through the professional organization, participates in creating a positive practice environment and maintaining safe, equitable social and economic working conditions in nursing.
- The nurse practices to sustain and protect the natural environment and is aware of its consequences on health.
- The nurse contributes to an ethical organizational environment and challenges unethical practices and settings.

4. Nurses and co-workers
    - The nurse sustains a collaborative and respectful relationship with co-workers in nursing and other fields.
    - The nurse takes appropriate action to safeguard individuals, families, and communities when their health is endangered by a co-worker or any other person.
    - The nurse takes appropriate action to support and guide co-workers to advance ethical conduct (ICN, 2–4).

As evident by the discussion in previous chapters in this text, nursing is guided not only by a code of ethics and standards of practice but also by theoretical concepts. The concepts that guide professional nursing practice fit the culture and need of a certain value structure.

Nursing Practice Influences in the United States

In the United States, nursing is a dynamic and progressive discipline with a deep concentration on practice, theory, and research. This complex triad of focus has developed nursing practice to a level that the Institute of Medicine (IOM) recommends nursing "practice to the full extent of their education and training" (2011). Many factors influence the practice of professional nursing; this chapter focuses on the Institute of Medicine recommendations, American Nurses Association Scope, and Standards and Caring.

Institute of Medicine Recommendations

Since the IOM's (2010) release of *The Future of Nursing: Leading Change, Advancing Health,* nursing has influenced U.S. policy changes in law and health care to provide nurses the legal support to advance practice and educate the public on the role of the nurse. This has also influenced the practice of nursing and the need to define the advancing role of the nurse and the advanced practice nurse. These IOM recommendations are intended to assist nurses in articulating the value provided to communities served by professional nurses. This report contains eight recommendations, all of which will promote nursing and advance clinical nursing practice to allow significant impacts on care delivery and patient outcomes. The IOM recommendations are as follows:

> *Recommendation 1: Remove scope-of-practice barriers.* Advance practice nurses should be able to practice to the full extent of their education and training (279).

Recommendation 2: Expand opportunities for nurses to lead and diffuse collaborative improvement efforts. Private and public funders, health care organizations, nursing education programs, and nursing associations should expand opportunities for nurses to lead and manage collaborative efforts with physicians and other members of the health care team to conduct research and to redesign and improve practice environments and health systems. These entities should also provide opportunities for nurses to diffuse successful practices (279).

Recommendation 3: Implement nurse residency programs. State boards of nursing, accrediting bodies, the federal government, and health care organizations should take actions to support nurses' completion of a transition-to-practice program (nurse residency) after they have completed a prelicensure or advanced practice degree program or when they are transitioning into new clinical practice areas (280).

Recommendation 4: Increase the proportion of nurses with a baccalaureate degree to 80% by 2020. Academic nurse leaders across all schools of nursing should work together to increase the proportion of nurses with a baccalaureate degree from 50 to 80 percent by 2020. These leaders should partner with education accrediting bodies, private and public funders, and employers to ensure funding, monitor progress, and increase the diversity of students to create a workforce prepared to meet the demands of diverse populations across the lifespan (280).

Recommendation 5: Double the number of nurses with a doctorate by 2020. Schools of nursing, with support from private and public funders, academic administrators and university trustees, and accrediting bodies, should double the number of nurses with a doctorate by 2020 to add to the cadre of nurse faculty and researchers, with attention to increasing diversity (281).

Recommendation 6: Ensure that nurses engage in lifelong learning. Accrediting bodies, schools of nursing, health care organizations, and continuing competency educators from multiple health professions should collaborate to ensure that nurses and nursing students and faculty continue their education and engage in lifelong learning to gain the competencies needed to provide care for diverse populations across the lifespan (282).

Recommendation 7: Prepare and enable nurses to lead change to advance health. Nurses, nursing education programs, and nursing associations should prepare the nursing workforce to assume leadership positions across all levels, while public, private, and governmental health care decision makers should ensure that leadership positions are available to and filled by nurses (283).

Recommendation 8: Build an infrastructure for the collection and analysis of interprofessional health care workforce data. The National Health Care Workforce Commission, with oversight from the Government Accountability Office and the Health Resources and Services Administration, should lead a collaborative effort to improve research and the collection and analysis of data on health care workforce requirements. The Workforce Commission and the Health Resources and Services Administration should collaborate with state licensing boards, state nursing workforce centers, and the Department of Labor in this effort to ensure that the data are timely and publicly accessible (284).

AMERICAN NURSES ASSOCIATION SCOPE AND STANDARDS OF PRACTICE

The largest impact on the clinical practice of professional nursing is the *ANA Scope and Standards of Practice* (ANA, 2010); the first six standards, known as the *Standards of Practice,* are essential to the clinical practice of nurses of all specialties and education levels. The standards are (1) assessment, (2) diagnosis, (3) outcome identification, (4) planning, (5) implementation, and (6) evaluation. Standards 7 through 16 known as the *Standards of Professional Performance* are (7) ethics, (8) education, (9) evidenced-based practice and research, (10) quality of practice, (11) communication, (12) leadership, (13) collaboration, (14) professional practice evaluation, (15) resource utilization, and (16) environmental health (ANA). All 16 standards shape professional nursing practice. This chapter focuses on the first six standards.

The first six standards mirror the nursing process and the scientific method that all professional nurses are expected to utilize to reach a well-developed clinical decision related to patient-centered care. The nursing process is not linear or unidirectional but dynamic and flowing from one step to another as a starting point as a patient's health status changes. In addition, all registered nurses are to demonstrate competency in their professional roles in accordance to their educational level as defined by the standards.

Caring in Nursing Practice

The ANA greatly influences the practice of the clinical nurse in the United States: "The essence of nursing practice is caring" (ANA, 2010, 25). The organization has identified *caring* as the theoretical concept that guides nursing care in the United States and *caring behaviors* to be a central focus of professional nursing practice (Glembocki & Dunn, 2010). Watson, Swanson, and Koloroutis have contributed greatly to this body of knowledge.

Watson initially defined *caring* in nursing practice. Watson's model of human caring (1988) focused on the interpersonal relationship that is developed and occurs between patient and nurse. This model places the patient as the director of change and transformation of his or her healing and well-being. Healing occurs from within the patient, and the nurse facilitates, supports, and guides the transformations and changes.

Swanson (1991) expanded on Watson's model of human caring and developed five caring processes. They compose a method for nurses to put into practice the caring behaviors that facilitate transformation and change that patients will experience. The five processes are:

1. *Knowing*: Striving to understand an event as it has meaning in the life of the other
2. *Being with*: Being emotionally present to the other
3. *Doing for*: Doing for the other what she or he would do for herself or himself if it were possible.
4. *Enabling and informing*: Facilitating the other's passage through life transitions and unfamiliar events.
5. *Maintaining belief*: Maintaining belief in persons and their capacity to make it through events and transitions.

Swanson additionally identified caring behaviors that clinical nurses can use to implement each of the five processes into clinical practice.

Koloroutis (2004) developed the relationship-based care model, a holistic patient-centered model with six dimensions surrounding the central focus of the patient and family. The six dimensions are (1) leadership, (2) teamwork, (3) professional nursing, (4) care delivery, (5) resources, and (6) outcomes. Koloroutis also described three essential relationships: (1) of nurse with patients and families, (2) of nurse with self, and (3) of nurse with colleagues. The six dimensions and the three essential relationships provide the organizational structure for transformation of professional nursing practice.

Many hospitals in the United States use the patient-centered model, relationship-based care, to guide the clinical practice and nursing professionalism. The IOM (2011) has recommended that all hospitals practice a patient-centered model; relationship-based care is not only patient centered but promotes the growth and development of professional nursing.

GLOBAL NURSING ENVIRONMENT IN THE FUTURE

Professional nursing practice will remain in an eternal state of transformation as health care delivery and values and patient needs change to meet the demands and needs of all the world, not of only one country. Professional nursing has a valuable seat at the table for health care transformation and social justice. As clinical practice is influenced by the organizations that bring life and direction to nursing—the ICN, the IOM, and the ANA—nurses will continue to bring caring to every interaction with patients and families.

REFERENCES

American Nurses Association. (2010). *Scope and standards*. Silver Springs, MD: Author.

Glembocki, M. M., & Dunn, K. S. (2010). Building an organizational culture of caring: Caring perceptions enhanced with education. *The Journal of Continuing Education in Nursing, 41*(12), 565–570.

Institute of Medicine (IOM). (2011). *The future of nursing: Leading change, advancing health*. Washington, DC: National Academies Press.

International Council of Nurses. (2012). *The ICN code of ethics for nurses*. Geneva, Switzerland: Author.

International Council of Nurses. (2014). *Definition of nursing*. Geneva, Switzerland: Author.

Koloroutis, M. (Ed.). (2004). *Relationship-based care: A model for transforming practice*. Minneapolis, MN: Creative Health Care Management.

Manthey, M. (2002). *The practice of primary nursing* (2nd ed.). Minneapolis, MN: Creative Health Care Management.

Nightingale, F. (1936). *Notes on nursing: What it is and what it is not*. New York: D. Appleton & Co.

Swanson, K. (1991). Empirical development of a middle range theory of caring, *Nursing Research, 40*: 161–166.

Watson, J. (1988). New dimensions of human caring theory. *Nursing Science Quarterly, 1*(4), 75–181.

World Health Organization. (2011). *World Health Organization global health atlas*. Retrieved from http://apps.who.int/globalatlas/dataQuery/default.asp

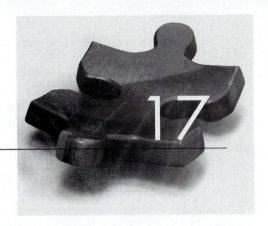

Nursing Conceptualizations from Around the World: Implications for Development of Global Nursing Theory and Research

Joyce J. Fitzpatrick

There is a remarkable consistency across the conceptualizations of nurses around the world. Nurse theorists clearly present their conceptual understandings focused on nursing interventions to enhance the health and wellness of individuals, families, and communities. Importantly, these same nurse theorists frame their work within the cultural environment in which they live and work. Thus, there are some cultural variations in emphasis and refinement of the core concepts with nursing's metaparadigm. Yet the similarities in conceptualizations place the discipline and its scholars in an important position for collaborative professional practice and scientific endeavors across geographic and cultural boundaries.

Our Australian colleagues have developed a conceptual model for the country that standardizes the conceptual framing of all nursing curricula. Professor White chaired the Australian Nursing and Midwifery Council (ANMAC) Accreditation Advisory Committee that developed the standards and describes not only the content but also the process that propelled this development. All professional nursing education in Australia is at the university level, and these new standards apply across all programs preparing professional nurses. Three of the nine standards that were developed are directly related to the conceptualization of nursing. These three standards delineate guidelines regarding the conceptual framework, program development and structure, and program content. White explicates the content of the Australian nursing standards within the context of the metaparadigm concepts of nursing. The environment encompasses all of Australia with a population of 23.5 million. Importantly, there is necessary attention to the multiculturalism and in particular, the indigenous populations, and, thus, cultural competence is a key component of nursing conceptualization. Health is conceptualized in relation to existing and emerging national and regional health priorities within the context of the World Health Organization's definition of health. The person is viewed as an active participant in his or her own care, and the family is defined as whatever the person names it to be. The nursing concept is highly developed in the Australian nursing standards, specifying not only the clinical skills of the professional nurses but also those for leadership and the management of others. Nursing is broader than the nurse–patient dyad and, according to White, encompasses a sociopolitical understanding of health, illness, health services, and policy.

Thus, in Australia, with the implementation of these new accreditation guidelines, there is great potential for expanding both the scientific knowledge undergirding the discipline and the clinical knowledge guiding professional nursing practice. Because these standards are newly enacted for accreditation, it will be important to track future progress of Australian nursing against these standards and in relation to global nursing developments. Particularly relevant will be the focus on cultural competence as the profession embraces global health issues and priorities.

In presenting a Canadian model of nursing, Dr. Gottlieb and Ms. Ponzoni focus on the positive nature of nursing; they describe a model of strength-based nursing as a shift away from the problem or deficit frame of reference that has often been described in nursing conceptualizations. Key values that guide this model include health and healing; uniqueness; holism and embodiment; subjective reality and created meaning; person-environment; learning, readiness, and timing; and collaborative partnerships. The authors' model further defines the nine characteristics of strengths, a concept that is important for both the professionals and for the recipients of care. Empowerment is central to strength-based nursing.

The authors of the strength-based model consider it an important deviation from other nursing models and define the metaparadigm concepts in positive empowering and enabling terms. For example, health is described as becoming, a process by which one creates wholeness and integration of self. Persons are defined as unique and capable of learning as well as having self-determination. Individuals create their own meaning of health and healing. Furthermore, person and environment are integral; they shape each other. The person experiences her or his environment in subjective ways and assigns meaning to this experience. Gottlieb and Ponzoni describe the nurse's obligation to society and the primary responsibility to help others create health and wholeness. Nurses must develop their own strengths of mindset, knowledge, relationship, and advocacy.

Gottlieb and Ponzoni connect their conceptualization to the work of Nightingale and propel us to consider a positive disciplinary model of nursing. This disciplinary perspective would help revise the labels used in our theoretical and professional practice knowledge development and would empower nurses to create a new reality from this perspective.

The Irish model of nursing presented by Professor McCarthy and Dr. Landers is a model of personhood that maintains the Irish cultural heritage values. The model is embedded in the cultural context of Celtic society, Irish language and customs, and the Catholic religion. Core concepts of personhood are soul friend, spirit, caring, love, and hope. The authors describe the nurse as a sensing individual, self-aware, knowledgeable, and present in nursing deliberations to enhance the nurse–patient relationship. The person, the recipient of care, is conceptualized with spiritual, biological, emotional, and sociological dimensions. Particular emphasis is given to the soul of the individual as the human body is conceptualized as an expression of the soul.

Each professional nurse is expected to understand the therapeutic effect of a caring environment and to facilitate development of a positive environment for health and healing. The goal of nursing is to assist others to achieve a sense of wellness and a positive movement from illness to health when illness is presented. The nurse acts as soul friend (teacher, companion, and spiritual guide) in helping the person transition to health and wellness.

The Irish theorists link their model of personhood to the caring theories of other nurse theorists. Hope and spirituality are positive forces within the nursing repertoire and guide nursing actions to move all individuals toward health. This model reflects a positive conceptualization, yet it bridges the gap between illness and a high level of wellness because the nurse must meet the person where he or she is on life's continuum of health and illness. The holistic nature of the conceptualization instructs us to expand the broader conceptualization of both our scientific and clinical knowledge development. And although the model is presented within the context of Irish culture and society, it would be expected that the nurse would necessarily be culturally aware as the society changes and becomes more diverse.

Professor Zanotti presents an Italian conceptualization of nursing as a stimulus of health-harmony drawing on the foundation of self-regulating and feedback processes to connect dimensions of biologic and cognitive domains with behavior. Persons are understood as having great capacity for deriving meaning and achieving health and harmony. Nurses help persons effect change in their lives through functional and behavioral interventions. Persons are viewed as dynamic systems, constantly constructing and restructuring their interactions with their environments. Persons are capable and aware and construct a subjective reality of the world in which they live.

Health within this Italian conceptualization emerges from the dynamic interactions of persons with their environments; health is a quality that reflects the person's capacity to control and modulate biological factors as well as cognitive and interpretive processes and to balance these with the person's energy reserves. The environment influences the person's health and harmony, and the professional nurse's role is to help the person modulate her or his health and harmony. Within this model, the professional nurse's role is limited if the person does not actively participate in her or his own movement toward health and harmony.

Nursing science and professional practice have been guided by this conceptualization of nursing. Instruments have been developed to guide research and practice, particularly on the assessment of health potential of individuals and the effectiveness of clinical nursing interventions to help individuals to achieve health and harmony. The focus on health and harmony is consistent with a positive definition of persons and their health; the active interventions of nurses to affect change in a person's health and harmony also support a broad and positive conceptualization of nursing.

Our colleague from Japan, Professor Yamauchi, describes a focused theoretical perspective, one targeting the area of physical assessment. Yamauchi asserts that nursing practice is grounded in excellent assessment skills, the ability to separate and understand, to make order out of chaos. Based on this skill, professional nurses are then prepared to both monitor and intervene. Nurses are expected to use their skills wherever patients are, particularly in clinical areas. One of the most important expectations of nurses is their ability to prioritize the care that should be provided. The nurse needs to understand what Yamauchi refers to as a "layered model of living functions," assessing the physical functions first and then the mental and social aspects that influence health. Through this assessment and priority-setting process, the nurse gains an understanding of the severity of the patient's condition, the stage of illness, and the frequency of the patient's response.

Professor Yamauchi's perspective on nursing has been implemented in nursing education in Japan and other Asian countries. This layered model of living functions serves as a very specific guide to nursing education, professional practice, and research. Although the model is specific in that it addresses the primary relationship between a nurse and a patient who presents with an illness or health problem, it is possible to extend this understanding to the broader context of nursing interventions to improve health and wellness.

In Spain under the leadership of the head of nursing at Barcelona's Clinic Hospital (BCH), Dr. Zabalegui developed a distinct model of nursing to guide professional practice, education, and research. This development was initiated by challenging nurses to describe the quality care that they provide and to articulate their vision of quality care. The nursing staff was driven to become a model of care for a high-complexity tertiary care and community hospital. Principles of nursing care that are explicit in the BCH model are patient empowerment, use of evidence-based best practices, effective communication with all members of the health care team, enhancement of the nurses' professional competence, and implementation of advanced practice and nursing leadership roles.

The BCH model defines the person, the recipient of care, as a biological, psychological, social, cultural, and spiritual being who collaborates to the extent possible in his or her own care. Nurses contribute to health (a dynamic, continuous process of balance and adaptation) through health promotion and attention to the well-being and quality of life of individuals, the family, and the community. Reflecting on the core principle of patient empowerment, the nurse facilitates the patient's involvement in care, encouraging self-care and development of increased knowledge of health and wellness. Implementation of the BCH model is reflected in the strategic plan for 2010–2015 with consistent structures and processes in place to enable nurses at BCH to function at the highest level of professional nursing. Whereas the model has been developed specifically for hospital-based nursing, it has components that can be translated to nursing practice, education, and research across settings. Furthermore, there are cross-country collaborations in place that will facilitate expansion and future dissemination of this BCH model.

Professor Kim has developed a theory of interpersonal caring that guides professional nursing practice, education, and research. The Kim model of interpersonal caring is closely linked to Dr. Kim's own religious beliefs and her lifelong commitment to serve people in need, especially those with mental health challenges and those who are underserved. Through the first nursing project worldwide to be funded through the United Nations Development Program, Dr. Kim demonstrated that individuals with chronic mental illnesses could make significant contributions to society. This experience led Dr. Kim to formalize her theory of interpersonal caring.

This interpersonal caring theory is focused on the goal of providing nurses and other caring professionals the disciplinary content to help patients realize their inner strengths and enhance their self-esteem and feelings of self-worth. Caring is defined as the primary focus of nursing, and interpersonal caring requires development of an interpersonal, therapeutic, compassion-based relationship between nurse and care receiver. The nurse–patient relationship is built on trust and respect, and nurse and care recipient are expected to collaborate to move toward identified health goals. Dr. Kim defines components of caring, including noticing, participating, sharing, active listening, companioning, complimenting, comforting, hoping, forgiving, and accepting. Each of these components of interpersonal caring is explicit and guides the nurse's actions in providing care. Furthermore, Dr. Kim describes persons as capable of self-actualization, a dynamic process that is enhanced through experiencing interpersonal caring. She defines health as a positive state characterized by knowledge, strength, will, and love for abundant life.

Although this theory of interpersonal caring grew from Dr. Kim's work with individuals with mental health challenges, it can be applied more broadly to all those cared for by nurses. Several applications of this theory can be expanded to guide clinical and scientific knowledge development for the discipline.

Person-centered nursing has been developed by Professor McCormack of the United Kingdom who has joined with his colleague, Professor McCance, to combine their theoretical perspectives, specifically the theoretical perspective of person-centered nursing practice with older persons, developed by their framework focused on patients' and nurses' caring. Thus, the person-centered nursing model is the synthesis of the two perspectives. Basic elements of this new model extend prior work. The core components of the theory are the attributes of the nurse, the care environment, the person-centered processes, and the expected outcomes as a result of effective person-centered care. The professional nurse is expected to be competent, committed, and possess self-knowledge, interpersonal skills, and clarity in values and beliefs. The care environment is one that is characterized by shared decision making and power sharing that has the potential for innovation and risk taking and yet is supportive. The focus of the interaction is on the person-centered processes that acknowledge the person's beliefs and values and are oriented to shared decision making and empowerment of the care recipient. The relationship is focused on holistic care that includes an expectation that the nurse has a sympathetic presence. The expected outcomes include the experience of good care, involvement in care, sense of well-being, and creation of a healthful environment.

The person-centered nursing model represents a broad conceptualization that has implications for the further extension for development of clinical and scientific knowledge in nursing. Its strength is the focus on specific interventions that are directly tied to health outcomes with the ultimate goal of enhancing human flourishing (i.e., growth for all involved in the therapeutic encounter). Health is conceptualized broadly within this model such that health reflects a positive life in all aspects of one's being.

These chapters describe conceptualizations developed by scholars in their own country, not in the United States. These included chapters from theorists in Australia, Canada, Ireland, Italy, Japan, Spain, South Korea, and the United Kingdom. A second set of chapters, those from authors in Egypt, Israel, Jordan, Mexico, and Thailand describe the status of theory development in their specific countries. Each of these authors identifies the need to adapt theories that are specific to the culture of his or her country and to extend theories that have been developed in the United States to be more consistent with the cultural differences.

Professors Abdelsalam and Mostafa from Egypt described the beginning state of theory use in their country, which is seen as a precursor to the development of theory. They present some specific examples of the use of theory to guide research. Theories used in the research examples provided are nursing theories developed by theorists in the United States (e.g., Orem, Peplau, and Roy) or adapted from other disciplines (e.g., psychology). Whereas there is beginning attention to theories guiding specific research projects, nursing theories have not thus far been used to guide nursing practice or nursing education in Egypt. The authors identify the potential for future developments concomitant with disciplinary development of nursing in the country.

Dr. Natan, Professor Ehrenfeld, and Dr. Itzhaki describe nursing in Israel as rooted in a unique religious, cultural, historic, and international political context, a situation that presents challenges for the development of both knowledge and professional practice. Emigration also presents particular challenges; most recently, there has been a substantial increase in nurses who emigrated from the former Soviet Union. In addition, the Israeli nursing population includes those Israeli citizens who are from the Arab minority in Israel. Nursing in Israel is widely influenced by Western culture, particularly that of the United States, and nursing education and practice are largely modeled accordingly. The authors believe that a transcultural nursing model is most appropriate to guide the development of the nursing discipline in Israel, particularly because the society is characterized by cultural diversity. Several research studies conducted by Israeli nurse scholars have been guided by transcultural nursing theories. In addition, professional nursing practice in Israel is focused on development of cultural competence, not only to provide better patient care but also to understand and relate to nursing colleagues from different cultural groups. There is increasing interest in further explication of the nursing discipline in Israel, including clinical and scientific knowledge development.

Professor Ahman and Ms. Dardas have described the aspiration of nurse leaders in Jordan to develop a culturally sensitive model to guide nursing knowledge development for theory, research, and professional practice. The authors note that theories developed in the Western world may not be congruent with Arab Muslim communities and note that more than 90% of Arabs are Muslim, and that Arabs are more homogenous than Westerners in their outlook on life. Thus, the authors identify the need for a culturally tailored nursing conceptualization for Arab nursing. Particularly important in the Arab Muslim culture, according to the authors, is a focus on spiritual wellness as a prerequisite for health of body and mind and a focus on the family rather than the individual as dominant, which is paramount in most Western models. Within the recent past, there have been major strides in the development of professional nursing education and professional practice in Jordan, and cultural competence is an important foundation for excellence. Thus, the authors identify the models of transcultural nursing that are most consistent with and have the potential for further adaptation to the Arab Muslim culture, including the religious teachings of Islam that are central to the culture and society and, thus, to nursing.

Professors Gallegos and Salazar describe the use of nursing theory in Mexico, including the adaptation of nursing theories from the United States and the application of theories primarily in research and education and, to a lesser extent, to guide nursing practice. Within the content of professional practice, the focus is primarily on the "doing" of nursing rather than on the development of the knowledge base for clinical interventions. Even so, the nursing care plans often have embedded within them a focus on enhancing self-care, a theoretical construct derived from the self-care model of nursing. The authors provide further evidence of the application of other models in nursing practice, most specifically those of Henderson and Orem. Nursing research in Mexico also is largely guided by the theories of Orem and Roy with a number of studies focused on various components of adaptation and self-care, including both descriptive and interventional studies. The particular investigators have delineated middle-range theories from these two models and have targeted persons with particular health challenges.

Importantly, the authors have noted the need for development of theories that are specific to their culture but also note that this might include further refinement of existing nursing theories.

Drs. Suwonnaroop, Piyopasakul, and Panitrat describe the development of nursing in Thailand; particularly relevant is the recent development of higher education with more than 60 university nursing schools, including master's and doctoral education. Nursing theory has been taught since 1977 and in 1987 became a core subject in university education at the lead university in Thailand. Nurses play a key role in primary health care in the country with a concomitant shift in perspective from illness care to health promotion. Thus far, Western nursing theories have been used to guide nursing practice and science in Thailand, including the nursing theories of Orem, Pender, and Roy and the adaptation of theories from social psychology. With a renewed emphasis on health care reform in Thailand, there is an identified need to formalize nursing knowledge development and explicate the contributions to clinical and scientific work of nurses with particular attention to the complexity of the current health care needs of the country.

As reflected in much of this text, nursing theory is in the early stages of development. Much of the theory development work that began in the United States in the 1970s has influenced the conceptualizations of nurse scholars from around the world, particularly of these nurses who received their doctoral education in the United States. Often these scholars have returned to their home countries and refined the U.S.-based theories to fit the sociocultural dimensions of their nursing world and work. Most important here is to acknowledge the similarities and consistencies across the nursing conceptualizations, independent of country of origin. This finding augers well for the future development of nursing science to guide professional practice.

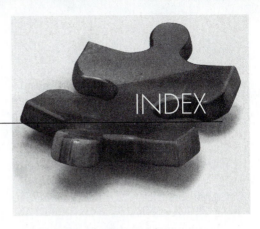
INDEX

Note: Page numbers with *f* indicate figures; those with *t* indicate tables.